MW01253101

Football and Health Improvement: An Emergent Field

There is developing interest in the use of sporting settings as a channel to connect people to health improvement services, and an emerging body of research highlights football as being associated with positive motivational and social elements that support the maintenance of a physically active lifestyle. This book provides insights into a range of issues surrounding the role of football as a vehicle for health improvement for different groups.

The contributors to this volume share some of the challenges and the benefits of using professional football settings as a channel for connecting people to health improvement opportunities. These chapters will be of interest to a range of stakeholders involved in research, policy and practice who stand to benefit from building partnerships with colleagues with expertise in (1) conducting evaluation and (2) reporting evaluation and research outcomes in peer-reviewed mediums, reflecting the value of partnerships between football-led health improvement and evaluators. This book was originally published as a special issue of *Soccer & Society*.

Daniel Parnell is a Senior Lecturer in Business Management at Manchester Metropolitan University, UK. His research interests cover the sport and leisure sectors within the United Kingdom and he works globally on a number of projects, in particular on the social role of sport.

Andy Pringle is a Reader in Physical Activity, Exercise and Health at Leeds Beckett University, UK. He researches the impact of physical activity and public health interventions. He is 'Fellow' of the Royal Society of Public Health and a Topic Expert (in 'physical activity') for the National Institute of Health and Care Excellence.

Football and Health Improvement: An Emergent Field

Edited by
Daniel Parnell and Andy Pringle

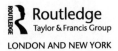

Routledge
Taylor & Francis Group

LONDON AND NEW YORK

First published 2017
by Routledge
2 Park Square, Milton Park, Abingdon, Oxon, OX14 4RN, UK

and by Routledge
711 Third Avenue, New York, NY 10017, USA

Routledge is an imprint of the Taylor & Francis Group, an informa business

© 2017 Taylor & Francis

British Library Cataloguing in Publication Data
A catalogue record for this book is available from the British Library

ISBN 13: 978-1-138-22146-8

Typeset in TimesNewRomanPS
by diacriTech, Chennai

Publisher's Note
The publisher accepts responsibility for any inconsistencies that may have arisen during the conversion of this book from journal articles to book chapters, namely the possible inclusion of journal terminology.

Disclaimer
Every effort has been made to contact copyright holders for their permission to reprint material in this book. The publishers would be grateful to hear from any copyright holder who is not here acknowledged and will undertake to rectify any errors or omissions in future editions of this book.

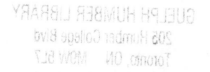

Contents

CONTENTS

Citation Information

The chapters in this book were originally published in the journal *Soccer & Society*, volume 17, issue 2 (March 2016). When citing this material, please use the original page numbering for each article, as follows:

Chapter 1
Football and health improvement: an emerging field
Daniel Parnell and Andy Pringle
Soccer & Society, volume 17, issue 2 (March 2016) pp. 171–174

Chapter 2
A perspective from key stakeholders on football and health improvement
Angus Martin, Simon Morgan, Daniel Parnell, Matthew Philpott, Andy Pringle, Michael Rigby, Andy Taylor and Jon Topham
Soccer & Society, volume 17, issue 2 (March 2016) pp. 175–182

Chapter 3
Supporting lifestyle risk reduction: promoting men's health through professional football
S. Zwolinsky, J. McKenna, A. Pringle, A. Daly-Smith, S. Robertson and A. White
Soccer & Society, volume 17, issue 2 (March 2016) pp. 183–195

Chapter 4
Effectiveness of a community football programme on improving physiological markers of health in a hard-to-reach male population: the role of exercise intensity
Andrew Thomas Hulton, David Flower, Rebecca Murphy, Dave Richardson, Barry Drust and Kathryn Curran
Soccer & Society, volume 17, issue 2 (March 2016) pp. 196–208

Chapter 5
Evaluating conflict mitigation and health improvement through soccer: a two-year study of Mifalot's 'United Soccer for Peace' programme
Tal Litvak-Hirsch, Yair Galily and Michael Leitner
Soccer & Society, volume 17, issue 2 (March 2016) pp. 209–224

Chapter 6

The pursuit of lifelong participation: the role of professional football clubs in the delivery of physical education and school sport in England
Daniel Parnell, Sarah Buxton, Des Hewitt, Matthew J. Reeves, Ed Cope and Richard Bailey
Soccer & Society, volume 17, issue 2 (March 2016) pp. 225–241

Chapter 7

Can 'English Premier League' funding for PE and school sport achieve its aims?
Stephen Zwolinsky, Jim McKenna, Daniel Parnell and Andy Pringle
Soccer & Society, volume 17, issue 2 (March 2016) pp. 242–245

Chapter 8

The influence of club football on children's daily physical activity
Glen Nielsen, Anna Bugge and Lars Bo Andersen
Soccer & Society, volume 17, issue 2 (March 2016) pp. 246–258

Chapter 9

Football for health: getting strategic
Simon Lansley and Daniel Parnell
Soccer & Society, volume 17, issue 2 (March 2016) pp. 259–266

For any permission-related enquiries please visit:
http://www.tandfonline.com/page/help/permissions

Football and health improvement: an emerging field

Daniel Parnell[1] and Andy Pringle

Centre for Active Lifestyles, Research Institute for Sport, Physical Activity and Leisure, Leeds Beckett University, Leeds, UK

Less than 40% of men and 30% of women met the current recommendations for an active lifestyle and with insufficient physical activity levels, concerns prevail over the health and well-being of the UK population, along with thoughts as to how best to intervene.[1] There is developing interest in the use of sporting settings as a channel to connect people to health improvement services including Rugby League and Cricket.[2] While 'top flight' football clubs have also been deployed as a way for connecting to communities on health-related matters including those hard-to-engage groups from children to older adults.[3] An emerging body of research highlights football is associated with positive motivational and social elements that support the maintenance of a physically active lifestyle.[4]

Building on this interest, there has been substantial research output focused on football and health promotion. For instance, in a major development, researchers in Scotland recently shared clinically significant outcomes emerging from an RCT which assessed the impact of a gender sensitized weight management programme for men delivered in/by the Scottish Premier League.[5] Whilst, Bangsbo and colleagues continued their 'outstanding' research building upon the evidence of how football can support the treatment and management of a range of diseases across the lifespan.[6] Reflecting the diversity of research designs, which are deployed to assess the impact of interventions, a special issue on Football and Inclusivity was published in 2014 and highlighted the role of football in delivering a range of social- and lifestyle-related behaviours and conditions.[7] In our own Institution, colleagues at Leeds Beckett University have continued to report the impact of football-led health improvement in a range of settings across the adult lifespan including men and older adults.[8]

Football and health improvement: this special issue

We are delighted to bring an eclectic mix of original studies and reflective accounts from colleagues. We anticipate that these contributions will be of interest to a range of stakeholders involved in research, policy and practice. With those thoughts in mind, we start with an 'Applied Editorial' from colleagues from the fields of both

---

[1]Current affiliation: Faculty of Business and Law, Business in Sport, Centre for Business and Society, Business School, Manchester Metropolitan University, UK.

Football and Health. In doing so, contributors share some of the challenges and the benefits of using professional football settings as a channel for connecting people to health improvement opportunities. In the understanding that football has been used to connect with hard-to-engage populations, Zwolinsky's paper reports further outcomes from a gender-specific health promotion programme for men delivered in Championship and Premier League Football Clubs. Within the same national men's health programme, Hulton and Colleague's demonstrate how physiological markers have been to assess health effects with a hard-to-reach male population within one specific club. The First World War Christmas Day ceasefire is 'perhaps' one of the most commonly cited examples of how football has been used to build relations during conflict situations, albeit temporarily. In a different context, Tal and colleagues paper evaluating conflict mitigation and health improvement through football, offers an interesting contribution of how sport is being deployed to build community relations and resolve conflict. Guidance on evaluation advises that programme evaluations should not only assess impact, but also the process of delivery,[9] Parnell and colleagues paper provides applied insights from football and school practitioners who delivered an extended physical education and school sport programme to develop lifelong participation in children/young people across primary schools. Zwolinsky and colleagues offer a short communication on the role of professional football clubs in the delivery of physical education and school sport. This line of interest in children's activity continues through Nielsen and colleagues article that explores the influence of club football and school recess activity on overall physical activity levels of Danish children. Such contributions are an important part of well-rounded evaluations that provide the perspectives of a range of stakeholders when shaping future provisions. We have also been encouraged by critical reflections of practitioners on this special issue. Indeed, Lansley's paper reflects the economic and policy debates of using sports-based intervention for health promotion. In preparing this compilation of papers, we have encountered practitioners who stand to benefit from building partnerships with colleagues with expertise in (I) conducting evaluation and (II) reporting evaluation and research outcomes in peer-reviewed mediums, reflecting the value of partnerships between football-led health improvement and evaluators.[10] In preparing this special issue, we thank all who engaged with the call for papers. We hope that the offerings included in this issue will create interest and provoke both discussion and dialogue in shaping programme implementation, research and evaluation.

Notes

1. The Information Centre for Health and Social Care, 'Statistics on Obesity'; Pringle et al., 'Health Improvement and Professional Football: Players on the Same Side'.
2. Pringle et al., 'Effect of a National Programme of Men's Health Delivered in English Premier League Football Clubs'; Triveldy, 'Oral Health Through Sport'; and Witty and White, 'Tackling Men's Health: Implementation of a Male Health Service in a Rugby Stadium'.
3. Parnell et al., 'Football in the Community Schemes: Exploring the Effectiveness of an Intervention in Promoting Positive Healthful Behaviour Change'; Parnell et al., 'Reaching Older People with Physical Activity Delivered in Football Clubs: The Reach, Adoption and Implementation Characteristics of the Extra Time Programme'.
4. Krustrup et al., 'Recreational Football as a Health Promoting Activity: A Topical Review'; Parnell and Richardson, 'Introduction: Football and Inclusivity'.

5. Hunt et al., 'A Gender-sensitised Weight Loss and Healthy Living programme for Overweight and Obese Men Delivered by Scottish Premier League Football Clubs (FFIT): A Pragmatic Randomised Controlled Trial'.
6. Bangsbo, Krustrup, and Dvorak, 'Special Issue: Football for Health – Prevention and Treatment of Non-communicable Diseases across the Lifespan through Football'.
7. Parnell and Richardson, 'Introduction: Football and Inclusivity'; Bingham et al., 'Fit Fans: Perspectives of a Practitioner and Understanding Participant Health Needs within a Health Promotion Programme for Older Men Delivered within an English Premier League Football Club'; Curran et al., 'Ethnographic Engagement from within a Football in the Community Programme at an English Premier League Football Club'; Pringle et al., 'Effect of a Health-improvement Pilot Programme for Older Adults Delivered by a Professional Football Club: The Burton Albion Case Study'; and Rutherford et al., '"Motivate": The Effect of a Football in the Community Delivered Weight Loss Programme on over 35-year Old Men and Women's Cardiovascular Risk Factors'.
8. Parnell et al. 'Reaching Older People with Physical Activity Delivered in Football Clubs: The Reach, Adoption and Implementation Characteristics of the Extra Time Programme'; Pringle et al., 'Effect of a National Programme of Men's Health Delivered in English Premier League Football Clubs'.
9. Dugdill and Stratton, *Evaluating Sport and Physical Activity Interventions: A Guide for Practitioners.*
10. Parnell et al., 'Understanding Football as a Vehicle for Enhancing Social Inclusion: Using an Intervention Mapping Framework'.

References

Bangsbo, J., P. Krustrup, and J. Dvorak. 'Special Issue: Football for Health – Prevention and Treatment of Non-communicable Diseases across the Lifespan through Football'. *Scandinavian Journal of Medicine & Science in Sport* 24, S1 (2014): 1–150.

Bingham, D.D., D. Parnell, K. Curran, R. Jones, and D. Richardson. 'Fit Fans: Perspectives of a Practitioner and Understanding Participant Health Needs within a Health Promotion Programme for Older Men Delivered within an English Premier League Football Club'. *Soccer & Society* 15, no. 6 (2014): 883–901.

Curran, K., D. Bingham, D. Richardson, and D. Parnell. 'Ethnographic Engagement from within a Football in the Community Programme at an English Premier League Football Club'. *Soccer & Society* 15 (2014): 934–50.

Dugdill, L., and G. Stratton. *Evaluating Sport and Physical Activity Interventions: A Guide for Practitioners.* University of Salford, 2013. http://usir.salford.ac.uk/3148/1/Dugdill_and_Stratton_2007.pdf (accessed September 24, 2013).

Dunn, K., B. Drust, D. Flower, and D. Richardson. 'Kicking the Habit: A Bio-psychosocial Account of Engaging Men Recovering from Drug Misuse in Recreational Football'. *Journal of Men's Health* 8 (2011): 233.

Hunt, K., S. Wyke, C. Gray, A. Anderson, A. Brady, C. Bunn, P.T. Donnon, et al. 'A Gender-sensitised Weight Loss and Healthy Living Programme for Overweight and Obese Men Delivered by Scottish Premier League Football Clubs (FFIT): A Pragmatic Randomised Controlled Trial'. *The Lancet* 383 (2014): 1211–21.

Krustrup, P., P. Aagaard, L. Nybo, J. Petersen, M. Mohr, and J. Bangsbo. 'Recreational Football as a Health Promoting Activity: A Topical Review'. *Scandinavian Journal of Medicine & Science in Sports* 20 (2010): 1–13.

Parnell, D., A. Pringle, P. Widdop, and S. Zwolinsky. 'Understanding Football as a Vehicle for Enhancing Social Inclusion: Using an Intervention Mapping Framework'. *Social Inclusion* 3 (2015): 158–66.

Parnell, D., A. Pringle, S. Zwolinsky, J. McKenna, Z. Rutherford, D. Richardson, L. Trotter, M. Rigby, M.J. Hargreaves. 'Reaching Older People with Physical Activity Delivered in Football Clubs: The Reach, Adoption and Implementation Characteristics of the Extra Time Programme'. *BMC Public Health* 15 (2015). doi: 10.1186/s12889-015-1560-5. http://www.biomedcentral.com/1471-2458/15/220.

Parnell, D., G. Stratton, B. Drust, and D. Richardson. 'Football in the Community Schemes: Exploring the Effectiveness of an Intervention in Promoting Healthful Behaviour Change'. *Soccer & Society* 14 (2013): 35–51.

Pringle, A., J. McKenna, and S. Zwolinsky. 'Health Improvement and Professional Football: Players on the Same Side?' *Journal of Policy Research in Tourism Leisure and Events* 5 (2013): 207–12.

Pringle, A., D. Parnell, S. Zwolinsky, J. Hargreaves, and J. McKenna. 'Effect of a health improvement programme for older adults delivered in/by Burton Albion FC'. *Soccer & Society* 15, no. 6 (2014): 902–18.

Pringle, A., S. Zwolinsky, J. Hargreaves, L. Lozano, and J. McKenna. 'Assessing the Impact of Football-based Health Improvement Programmes: Stay Onside, Avoid Own Goals and Bag the Evaluation Net'. *Soccer & Society* 15, no. 6 (2014): 970–87.

Pringle, A., S. Zwolinsky, J. McKenna, A. Daly-Smith, S. Robertson, and A. White. 'Effect of a National Programme of Men's Health Delivered in English Premier League Football Clubs'. *Public Health* 127 (2013): 18–26.

Pringle, A., S. Zwolinsky, J. McKenna, A. Daly-Smith, S. Robertson, and A. White. 'Health Improvement for Men and Hard-to-Engage-Men Delivered in English Premier League Football Clubs'. *Health Education Research* 29, no. 3 (2014): 503–20.

Rutherford, Z., B. Gough, S. Seymour-Smith, C. Matthews, J. Wilcox and D. Parnell '"Motivate": The Effect of a Football in the Community Delivered Weight Loss Programme on over 35-Year Old Men and Women's Cardiovascular Risk Factors'. *Soccer & Society* 15 (2014): 951–69.

Trivedy, C. 'Oral Health through Sport'. *British Dental Journal* 210 (2011):150. http://www.nature.com/bdj/journal/v210/n4/full/sj.bdj.2011.98.html (accessed January 24, 2012).

Witty, K., and A. White. 'Tackling Men's Health: Implementation of a Male Health Service in a Rugby Stadium'. *Community Practitioner* 84 (2011): 29–32.

A perspective from key stakeholders on football and health improvement

Angus Martin[a], Simon Morgan[b], Daniel Parnell[c], Matthew Philpott[d], Andy Pringle[c], Michael Rigby[e], Andy Taylor[f] and Jon Topham[g]

[a]Football League Trust, Preston, UK; [b]Premier League, London, UK; [c]Centre for Active Lifestyles, Institute of Sport, Physical Activity and Leisure, Leeds Beckett University, Leeds, UK; [d]European Healthy Stadia Network CIC, Liverpool, UK; [e]Football Foundation, London, UK; [f]Burton Albion Community Trust, Burton on Trent, UK; [g]Public Health, Stafford, UK

Football is one of the most popular sports worldwide. Much of the research literature is primarily focused on contributions from the academic community. Given this, the Editors were motivated to provide an opportunity for practitioners and commissioners from applied settings to share their perspectives. This applied article offers insights from 'key players' activity involved in football-led health improvement interventions.

Introduction

Football has been highlighted as the most popular team sport in the world. Recently, an emerging body of the literature highlights football-led health improvement as a vehicle for positive changes in physical and social health impacts. This adds further weight to support the role of football in delivering success in a range of lifestyle-related behaviours and conditions across the lifespan.[1] The purpose of this special issue was to invite contributions on the role of football-led interventions and their impact on health improvement. In doing so, the Editors [Parnell and Pringle] seek to bring together current perspectives from key stakeholders in the area. Given that many literary contributions come from the academic community, the Editors were motivated to provide practitioners and commissioners as well as researchers with an opportunity to share their perspectives. As such, this editorial offers applied insights from 'key players' actively involved in football-led health improvement. Contributors will not only provide insight into the scope and reach of health improvement interventions, but also considerations for practitioners and researchers working in this area. In no hierarchical order, we are pleased that colleagues from the English Premier Football League, English Football League Trust, the Football Foundation, European Healthy Stadia Network, Burton Albion Football Club (Burton Albion Community Trust) and Staffordshire Public Health have joined us in providing this editorial.

Current affiliation: Faculty of Business and Law, Business in Sport, Centre for Business and Society, Business School, Manchester Metropolitan University, UK.

FOOTBALL AND HEALTH IMPROVEMENT: AN EMERGENT FIELD

The global brand of the English Premier League and the Football League is associated historically with football in England and with the local communities where many football clubs are positioned geographically. The English Premier League and Football League clubs have a long history of engagement with their local communities and all clubs have associated community foundations, which are often charities [with a number of exceptions who have charitable arms, but manage their community engagement activity as part of the club's internal corporate social responsibility function] that engage within their local communities delivering on a range of social agendas including education, social inclusion, crime reduction and health improvement. For many observers, the work undertaken within the community programmes of the professional football clubs in England is considered world leading. The first contributor is Mr Simon Morgan, Head of the English Premier League Charitable arm, who offers an update and insight into their work:

> The Premier League is one of the most popular and exciting sports competitions in the world. Off the field the Premier League has a huge commitment to social responsibility and supports Clubs in their important roles as hubs at the heart of their communities. This commitment includes building new grassroots facilities, providing activities to increase sporting participation and a focus on young people and education, particularly improving the quality of Physical Education (PE) sessions in schools. Football is also a key tool to promote health improvement. In recent years the Premier League has funded a men's health programme and a mental health programme with the outcomes proving that football clubs have a unique ability to engage with their local communities and provide social benefit to the participants.

> The Premier League is currently focusing its priority on young people and providing them access to high quality PE sessions in school and pathways into other inclusive sporting opportunities including competition. Clubs delivered over 66,000 h of fun PE lessons last year. By providing physical literacy and fundamental movement skills at an early age this will promote the healthy advantage of creating an active lifestyle.

> The biggest challenge is for the health sector to appreciate the important role the clubs can play in meeting their objectives. The clubs can engage hard to reach and inactive people that other organisations can't. The clubs are then able to provide bespoke programmes tailored to the individuals needs be they sport, exercise or re-engaging with the community. Similarly the importance of PE within a balanced national curriculum should not be underestimated and every child should have access to a high quality PE. This not only builds self-confidence but also is healthy and good for communities. The Premier League is keen to promote participation in sport from a young age and then help to keep them playing throughout their life regardless of economic or social background.

> Football, the Premier League and our clubs have an important role to play in helping to promote and develop a healthy lifestyle in young people and then to sustain them by providing pathways into sporting opportunities that suit them as individuals.

Football in England extends beyond the English Premier League; as previously mentioned The Football League plays an important role in reaching out across England and Wales geographically to deliver football-based health improvement through its 72 associated football clubs. As with the English Premier League, the Football League has a charitable and community-oriented operation committed to achieving football-related social objectives. Mr Angus Martin, Business Development Manager and Lead for Education at the Football League Trust:

> The Football League Trust is a registered charity, which acts as an umbrella organisation to support and represent the interests of a national network of charities housed within Football League clubs. This network engages with over 1.5 million individuals

each year across projects encompassing sport, health, education and inclusion. In simplest terms we use the power of sport to engage with people of all ages and backgrounds to engender positive community action.

Our trusts deliver a very wide range of health initiatives from within their respective football clubs. This includes everything from healthy eating projects in primary schools through to more challenging work with mental health. This extends to projects focused on particular groups of the population (such as women and girls, children and young people and older adults). There is also significant overlap between health projects and our other key areas of work – sport, education and inclusion. Using sport and football in particular we are able to engage with some of the hardest to reach people in our communities, working with them to both educate and inspire positive change.

The biggest challenge for us with regards to increasing the health improvement work that our trusts carry out is a combination of access to funding and also the awareness of health commissioners of the capabilities of our network. We work hard to capture the data behind successful projects we deliver to use this to build our argument to funders and also invest significant time and money into providing appropriate health-related continuing professional development and training for our staff.

Football and sport obviously isn't the whole answer to health improvement, but we certainly feel that we can play a significant part and we have a particular strength with regards to being able to engage with all areas of our communities. The use of our stadia and professional players as inspiring venues and positive role models is a further strength with regards to helping us achieve health improvements.

Facilities and stadia are both critically important features in football from a grassroots perspective through to the stadia of professional football clubs. Indeed, facilities and stadia each have a role to play in providing infrastructure, locations, facilities, and in some cases, cultural landmarks to deliver health-related messages, interventions and projects. With those thoughts in mind, the next contributor is, Mr Michael Rigby, Head of Information Systems and Business Intelligence for the Football Foundation. Michael offers his perspectives into the Football Foundation role in helping achieve more physically active populations through upgrading public sports facilities:

The UK has amongst the worst levels of obesity in Western Europe and it also has amongst the worst public sports facilities. Comparable countries like Germany, France and Holland provide excellent local sports facilities, yet Britain lacks these crucial venues that enable people to stay fit and healthy through playing regular sport.

We are therefore, as a country, effectively trying to combat obesity without a major tool in our armoury. This was underlined by independent research commissioned by the Football Foundation to establish how impactful third generation (3G) artificial grass pitches (AGP) are on the health of the people who use them.

The Football Foundation was founded by the Premier League, The FA (Football Association) and the Government in 2000 to improve grassroots facilities, and to get more people playing our national game. In the last 15 years the Foundation has awarded grants worth £513 m and multiplied our Funding Partners' investment by attracting an additional £730 m in partnership funding, which means more than £1.2 bn has been invested in the areas of most need and where it will have the most impact.

Investment has focused on the refurbishment of existing facilities and developing new ones, such as floodlit 3G AGPs and changing rooms, the Foundation has achieved substantial increases in participation. It has also improved the quality experience of players and helped achieve player retention at existing and new sites.

Last year the Foundation achieved an average increase in football participation of 11% at facilities that it invested in, compared to the level of football played at those sites the previous year. It also achieved a 25.8% increase across all sports, and has consistently managed to get local populations enjoying more regular physical activity each year. Achieved simply through expert targeting of investment and expanding the capacity and quality of the country's local sports infrastructure.

Furthermore, when asked to score out of five, with five being the most certain, if their health had improved as a result of playing on a 3G AGPs, 86% of the 274 players questioned gave an answer of between three and five – a strong indication that they felt 3G AGPs were contributing positively to their wellbeing.

Many of these 3G AGPs strengthen the connection between communities and their local professional club's community foundation who are delivering outreach work in some of the most deprived areas of the country. These types of programme are not only helping to keep people fit but also address mental health problems, such as depression and anxiety by providing self-esteem through increased social networks.

By providing more of these facilities the Foundation is ensuring that at least some of our population are able to avoid serious health issues like obesity, thus avoiding far more costly subsequent problems to their quality of life and to the National Health Service.

Addressing Public Health issues through football has grown in recent years,[2] especially through the development or redevelopment of new or existing facilities. Continuing the discussion on the role of facilities, it is pertinent to consider the broader role of sports stadia in delivering health improvement activities. Our next contributor is Dr Matthew Philpott, Director of the European Healthy Stadia Network CIC:

Football at recreational level is now well evidenced as an effective means of both preventing and treating non-communicable diseases.[3] There is also an increasing recognition of the role professional sports clubs, including football clubs, can play in improving the public health of local communities and those who interact with their sports venues. Building on European research carried out from 2007–2009,[4] the UK-based social enterprise European Healthy Stadia Network (hereon Healthy Stadia) works with professional sports clubs and governing bodies of sport to develop stadia as 'health promoting settings', offering assistance through guidance documents, case studies of good practice, benchmarking tools and research.

This settings-based approach emphasises the potential for sports venues to develop policies and interventions promoting healthier lifestyles across three cross-cutting themes: healthier stadium environments for fans and non-match day visitors (e.g. healthier food options); healthier club workforces (e.g. annual health checks); and, healthier populations in local communities (e.g. men's weight loss programmes). The most obvious of these categories to have developed over recent years has been the increase of community health interventions delivered by football clubs (predominantly based in Northern Europe). Such interventions have addressed a wide array of public health concerns (e.g. physical activity, healthier eating, and mental health) of which there are now a growing number of independently evaluated projects and randomised control trials.[5]

Although less visible, there has also been positive changes concerning health promoting policies and operations at football stadia and major sports events, in particular concerning tobacco and alcohol control, healthier eating options at catering outlets, active travel (walking and cycling to stadia), and the community use of club training and exercise facilities. Whilst it may come as a surprise that only 10 out of 54 national football associations in Europe have a coverall smoke-free policy,[6] it is promising that two of football's key governing bodies – FIFA and UEFA – have declared a ban on use and sale of tobacco at recent editions of their flagship international tournaments. Progress has also been made at club level in terms of healthier catering options such as low-calorie menus, healthier reformulation of traditional choices (e.g. use of low fat and low salt pastry), and supply of free drinking water, whilst clubs are increasingly investing in active travel assets such as bike locking racks, with KAA Gent in Belgium having now installed 3438 locking points at their 20,000 capacity stadium.

Health promoting stadium initiatives face a number of challenges, in particular over-coming the conflicting commercial and (in some cases) political concerns of clubs and governing bodies, but also problems of evaluating their overall impact on health – a common problem associated with population-based approaches to public health. There is also an argument that since the proliferation of healthy lifestyle projects delivered by 'arm's length' community foundations or trusts, some of the impetus for clubs them-selves to develop health promoting stadium initiatives has been downgraded, thereby disrupting the holistic concept of a health promoting club and stadium.

As the health and economic consequences of non-communicable diseases increases in Europe year upon year, there are still huge opportunities for football clubs to become *exemplar* health settings for certain population groups, something they are uniquely positioned to realise owing to fan loyalty, communications reach, and provision of specialist facilities.

The scope of contributions thus far highlights the potential of football-led health improvement to play a role in tackling non-communicable diseases. The English Premier League and Football League Trust outline the reach and scope of football organizations within England and Wales, whilst the Football Foundation and Healthy Stadia display the current potential of facilities and stadia. Our contributors endorse the role of football in contributing to Public Health outcomes. The focus of our editorial now shifts slightly as we consider the perspective of colleagues involved in commissioning and providing football-led health improvement at the front line! Mr Jon Topham, Locality Public Health Partnerships and Commissioning Lead for Public Health Staffordshire in the English East Midlands and collaborator Mr Andy Taylor, Head of Community at Burton Albion Community Trust (BACT). BACT is the community arm of Burton Albion Football Club and are part of the Football League Trust:

BACT is the charitable arm of Burton Albion Football Club and has been operating since September 2010, delivering a wide range of projects across the themes of Sport Participation, Education, Social Inclusion, Disability and Health. The engagement is part of a 'whole family' approach with delivery across the lifespan (from ages 2 to 80). Such engagement is delivered via targeted provision as a result of strong partner-ships and an innovative workforce consisting of family support workers, officers and practitioners.

BACT has worked closely with the local Public Health Commissioner and researchers specifically collaborator Dan Parnell (Leeds Beckett University) to design and deliver projects utilising the brand of Burton Albion Football Club to impact on the wider health agenda.[7] It is our belief, which is backed up by our increasing community engagement, that football clubs have a pivotal role to play in inspiring people of all ages to make positive life choices.

Within the last twelve months we have seen funded health projects such as Golden Goal (Over 50s Physical and Social Activity Club)[8] Head for Goal (Mental Health Football), Male Fit Fans (Bespoke men's health programme) emerge as sustainable models of provision. Current projects also include collaborations with East Stafford-shire Citizen Advice Bureau (Focussed on schools and families, projects not only help to promote lifestyle change but also help with home budgeting and money manage-ment. All projects offer participants pathways owing to the wide menu of programmes we currently deliver, ranging from the initial engagement through to volunteering and education programmes.

We believe that, as an agent for positive health changes, football clubs provide a base that is firmly rooted in the community; football clubs are not burdened with statutory baggage and provide a safe environment to effect 'change' in both fans and local communities. In the case of BACT, proactive engagement with all local partners a commitment to partnership working and a 'can-do' attitude have been at the heart of successful projects delivered in East Staffordshire.

This approach to partnership working, using the hook of football, to drive positive health change, does offer clear opportunities to reach particular groups of people, notably men and disaffected groups more generally. This is why BACT have worked in collaboration with Public Health on wider campaigns, for example the annual Health and Wellbeing fixture, which allows partner organisations to raise awareness of issues such as smoking, alcohol consumption, as well as health tests for the fans. The fan base of a football club (typically male) creates opportunities for partner organisations to engage with those harder to reach groups. This includes those individuals who may not go into a GP surgery for a health check or attend a local gym, but will engage with BAFC branded programmes and their staff.

It is important to set these achievements against the challenges facing football and community trusts/charities working within football clubs to meet the Public Health agenda. These include the following:

(1) Organizational buy in from the football club to the community trust/charity, which is critical. In the case of Burton Albion, the club is wholeheartedly supportive and this has enabled the BACT to flourish and to explore new ways of working.
(2) Recruiting the right staff and skill set.
(3) Planning interventions so they have a strategic fit.
(4) Funding to adequately resource effective interventions and evaluation.
(5) Balance between commercial and social objectives.

BACT and Staffordshire Public Health believe that football clubs have a huge role to play in meeting Health Improvement outcomes, in partnership with wider organisations from both the public and voluntary sector. In the past football has played a peripheral role in health improvement. Moving forward, we believe that Footballs Clubs and Trusts can provide a vehicle for developing 'scaled up' health improvement interventions that offer reach into previously untapped communities and really start to offer positive support for people to consider their own lifestyles and to encourage a mass movement for change.

Concluding comments

Contributions from our colleagues illustrate the scope and breadth of activity ranging from national programmes to local interventions forming part of the strategic context for health improvement. While these accounts are closely aligned to the emerging evidence supporting the impact of interventions, our contributors point out that effective intervention is not a given! Amongst other challenges, the need for, good planning, fidelity with local health priorities and effective collaborations are important in providing interventions that meet the health needs of participants. Increasing stakeholder awareness of the unique reach that football and football-led health improvement can playing meeting local health priorities will continue to be important. In doing so, well-designed monitoring and evaluation of programmes are essential in identifying which interventions are effective along with processes underlying these impacts.

Disclosure statement

No potential conflict of interest was reported by the authors.

Notes

1. Pringle et al., 'Health Improvement for Men and Hard-to-engage-men Delivered in English Premier League Football Clubs'; Parnell and Richardson, 'Introduction: Football and Inclusivity'; Hunt et al., 'A Gender-sensitised Weight Loss and Healthy Living Programme for Overweight and Obese men Delivered by Scottish Premier League Football Clubs (FFIT): A Pragmatic Randomised Controlled Trial'; Bangsbo, Krustrup, and Dvorák, 'Special Issue: Football for Health – Prevention and Treatment of Non-communicable Diseases across the Lifespan through Football'; and Parnell et al., 'Reaching Older People with PA Delivered in Football Clubs: The Reach, Adoption and Implementation Characteristics of the Extra Time Programme'.
2. Pringle et al., 'Health Improvement for Men and Hard-to-engage-men Delivered in English Premier League Football Clubs'; Parnell and Richardson, 'Introduction: Football and Inclusivity'; and Parnell et al., 'Reaching Older People with PA Delivered in Football Clubs: The Reach, Adoption and Implementation Characteristics of the Extra Time Programme'.
3. Bangsbo, Krustrup, and Dvorák, 'Special Issue: Football for Health – Prevention and Treatment of Non-communicable Diseases across the Lifespan through Football'.
4. Drygas et al., 'Good Practices and Health Policy Analysis in European Sports Stadia: Results from the "Healthy Stadia" Project'.
5. Hunt et al., 'A Gender-sensitised Weight Loss and Healthy Living Programme for Overweight and Obese Men Delivered by Scottish Premier League Football Clubs (FFIT): A Pragmatic Randomised Controlled Trial'; Dubuy et al., 'Evaluation of a Real World Intervention Using Professional Football Players to Promote a Healthy Diet and Physical Activity in Children and Adolescents from a Lower Socio-economic Background: A Controlled Pretest–posttest Design'; and Zwolinsky et al., 'Optimizing Lifestyles for Men Regarded as "Hard-to-reach" through Top-flight Football/Soccer Clubs'.
6. Healthy Stadia, *Survey of Smoke-free Policies at Football Stadia in Europe*.
7. Pringle et al. 'Effect of a Health-improvement Pilot Programme for Older Adults Delivered by a Professional Football Club: The Burton Albion Case Study'; Parnell et al., 'Understanding Football as a Vehicle for Enhancing Social Inclusion: Using an Intervention Mapping Framework'.
8. Pringle et al. 'Effect of a Health-improvement Pilot Programme for Older Adults Delivered by a Professional Football Club: The Burton Albion Case Study'.

References

Bangsbo, J., P. Krustrup, and J. Dvorák. 'Special Issue: Football for Health – Prevention and Treatment of Non-communicable Diseases across the Lifespan through Football. This Supplement Was Supported by an Unrestricted Educational Grant from Fédération Internationale de Football Association'. *Scandinavian Journal of Medicine & Science in Sports* 24, S1 (2104): 1–150.
Drygas, W., J. Ruszkowska, M. Philpott, O. BjÖrkstrÖm, M. Parker, R. Ireland, and M. Tenconi. 'Good Practices and Health Policy Analysis in European Sports Stadia: Results from the "Healthy Stadia" Project'. *Health Promotion International* 28, no. 2 (2013): 157–65.
Dubuy. V., L. De Cocker, I. De Bourdeaudhuij, L. Maes, J. Seghers, J. Lefevre, and G. Cardon. 'Evaluation of a Real World Intervention Using Professional Football Players to Promote a Healthy Diet and Physical Activity in Children and Adolescents from a Lower Socio-economic Background: A Controlled Pretest–Posttest Design'. *BMC Public Health* 14, no. 1 (2014): 457. http://www.biomedcentral.com/content/pdf/1471-2458-14-457.pdf.
Healthy Stadia. *Survey of Smoke-free Policies at Football Stadia in Europe*. 2015. http://www.healthystadia.eu/resource-library/tobacco-control/item/download/185_f431915daa4c05dd6a9592665b07790e.html (accessed January 10, 2015).

Hunt, K., S. Wyke, C.M. Gray, A.S. Anderson, A. Brady, C. Bunn, P.T. Donnan, et al. 'A Gender-sensitised Weight Loss and Healthy Living Programme for Overweight and Obese Men Delivered by Scottish Premier League Football Clubs (FFIT): A Pragmatic Randomised Controlled Trial'. *The Lancet* 383, (2014): 1211–21. doi: 10.1016/S0140-6736(13)62420-4.

Parnell, D., A. Pringle, J. McKenna, S. Zwolinsky, Z. Rutherford, J. Hargreaves, L. Trotter, M. Rigby, and D. Richardson. 'Reaching Older People with PA Delivered in Football Clubs: The Reach, Adoption and Implementation Characteristics of the Extra Time Programme'. *BMC Public Health* 15 (2015). http://www.biomedcentral.com/content/pdf/s12889-015-1560-5.pdf.

Parnell, D., A. Pringle, P. Widdop, and S. Zwolinsky. 'Understanding Football as a Vehicle for Enhancing Social Inclusion: Using an Intervention Mapping Framework'. *Social Inclusion* 3 (2015): 158–66.

Parnell, D., and D. Richardson. 'Introduction: Football and Inclusivity'. *Soccer & Society* 15, no. 6 (2014): 823–7.

Pringle, A., D. Parnell, S. Zwolinsky, J. Hargreaves, and J. McKenna. 'Effect of a Health-improvement Pilot Programme for Older Adults Delivered by a Professional Football Club: The Burton Albion Case Study'. *Soccer and Society* 15 (2014): 902–18.

Pringle, A., S. Zwolinsky, J. McKenna, S. Robertson, A. Daly-Smith, and A. White. 'Health Improvement for Men and Hard-to-engage-men Delivered in English Premier League Football Clubs'. *Health Education Research* 29 (2014): 503–20.

Zwolinsky, S., J. McKenna, A. Pringle, A. Daly-Smith, S. Robertson, and A. White. 'Optimizing Lifestyles for Men Regarded as 'Hard-to-Reach' through Top-Flight Football/Soccer Clubs'. *Health Education Research* 28, no. 3 (2013): 405–13. doi: 10.1093/her/cys108.

Supporting lifestyle risk reduction: promoting men's health through professional football

S. Zwolinsky[a], J. McKenna[a], A. Pringle[a], A. Daly-Smith[a], S. Robertson[b] and A. White[b]

[a]Centre for Active Lifestyles, Leeds Beckett University, Leeds, UK; [b]Centre for Men's Health, Leeds Beckett University, Leeds, UK

For men, unhealthy lifestyle behaviours including physical inactivity, a poor diet, smoking and excess alcohol represent major, modifiable causes of non-communicable disease worldwide. Innovative approaches that seek to overcome the barriers that men experience when attempting to deploy more self-care to manage these behaviours are required. This study assessed the outcomes of a 12-week men's health promotion intervention delivered in and by professional football clubs. Data comprised self-reports from 1667 men aged 18–75 years from 16 English Premier League and Championship football clubs. A multinomial logistic regression model estimated the probability of self-reporting a number of baseline lifestyle risk factors compared to a reference group with none. Wilcoxon signed-rank tests assessed differences in lifestyle risk profiles. Over 85% of participants presented with multiple risk factors. Men aged ≥35 years were least likely to present all four risk factors (OR: 0.45, 95% CI: 0.23–0.88), whereas unemployed men (OR: 3.64, 95% CI: 1.78–7.51) and those with no social support network (OR: 5.10, 95% CI: 2.44–10.50) were most likely to self-report all four lifestyle risks. The prevalence of risk factors was significantly reduced post-intervention ($z = -7.488$, $p < 0.001$, $r = -0.13$), indicating a positive effect, and potential public health significance. Findings show that men can respond positively to behaviourally-focused interventions delivered in familiar and local settings, like professional football clubs.

Introduction

The insidious nature of men's ill health is cause for concern in the UK and the whole of the European Union with the growing spectre of avoidable premature death and chronic disease.[1] Moreover, orthodox channels for health promotion are routinely ineffective for helping some groups of men to sustain lifestyle change.[2] Worse, the scarcity of evidence-based programmes that meet their needs means there is little opportunity for the refinement of existing practice.[3] Therefore, poor engagement and high attrition continue to characterize health interventions aimed at younger men, especially those delivered in community settings.[4] The combination of inadequate provision and challenging socio-economic circumstance heighten the prevalence of many avoidable health conditions.[5] Consequently, there is an urgent need to identify successful, replicable and innovative approaches for improving the health of men.[6]

Professional football settings can be effective at engaging men who are reluctant to seek help through conventional services.[7] Men can be difficult to attract into health improvement programmes, plus they have a reputation for neither initiating nor sustaining health modifying behaviour.[8] However, recent research investigating men's health in footballing contexts has shown positive effects for improving various cardiovascular markers and selected lifestyle behaviours. Men engaging exercise and diet programmes over a 10-week period demonstrated significant reductions in body weight, cholesterol and systolic blood pressure.[9] This weight loss was maintained over one year, well beyond the end of the programme. Further, in addition to well-established physiological benefits, the social experience of exercising can have positive benefits for mental health, including reducing depression,[10] social isolation and improving confidence.[11] These features often characterize groups of men considered harder-to-connect with that need the connection all-the-more.

Gender-sensitive interventions can play an important role in men's health. In part, this is because men are less likely than women to develop the helping social relationships that positively impact physical and mental health.[12] Since socially supportive networks and relationships operate behaviourally,[13] sporting and leisure contexts provide an interesting avenue for connecting with men over health and for constructing positive supportive links.[14] It is also clear that positive holistic health can be enhanced when interventions blend public health recommendations, provide increased social support and help participants to form strong and diverse natural social networks.[15] Improving these elements of social capital means that the prevalence of multiple lifestyle risk factors can also be reduced.[16] Leisure and sporting contexts have the potential to facilitate many of these attributes, therefore, overcoming determinants to engagement.

Unhealthy lifestyle behaviours including inactivity, poor diet, smoking and excess alcohol consumption increase the risk for non-communicable disease. Individually and collectively, they exact a huge toll on morbidity and mortality rates worldwide.[17] These four lifestyle risk factors are now emphasized by the UK National Health Service (NHS) in its Every Contact Counts policy,[18] and they underpin the 2020 impact goals for the US.[19] Although there has been a reported decline in the population displaying three or more lifestyle risk factors, this is mainly witnessed among those in higher socio-economic and educational groups.[20] The individual and combined prevalence of these risk factors confirms a non-random pattern of distribution across the population, especially among younger men, those in the lower social classes and with lower levels of education.[21] As a result, targeted health promotion interventions focusing on tangible short-term effects in at-risk groups are thought to be most effective.[22] Provisions within professional football clubs offer one possible way for overcoming many of the barriers that many men experience around attempting to deploy more self-care.

At present, there is a shortage of research investigating the prevalence and combinations of lifestyle risk factors in UK adults. Nevertheless, the available evidence serves to demonstrate the scale of the problem. Currently, it is estimated that around 60–70% of adult men present two or more of the big four lifestyle risk factors simultaneously.[23] However, eliminating these unhealthy behaviours could potentially reduce 74% of cardiovascular disease cases, 82% of coronary heart disease cases and 91% of diabetes cases.[24] Furthermore, the estimated benefit for those individuals who present zero compared to four lifestyle risk factors is equivalent to 14 years of extra life (when adjusted for gender, age, body mass index and socio-economic status).[25] With these thoughts in mind, this study aims to assess the most influential predictors of simultaneous lifestyle risk factors in men. It also aims to identify the outcomes of a 12-week health promotion intervention delivered in and by professional football clubs on reducing the prevalence of these risk factors.

Method

The intervention

'Premier League Health' (PLH) is a £1.63 m three year programme of men's health promotion delivered in and by professional football clubs.[26] This investment helped 16 English Premier League and Championship football clubs to promote men's health. These clubs are iconic, their histories and reputations are respected locally, while stadia are familiar and located in densely populated community settings. Men aged ≥18 years were recruited from community settings, drug and prison rehabilitation services, unemployment agencies and areas of low socio-economic status. Substantial training was provided to delivery staff around the contemporary understanding of behaviour change. Subsequently, staff at each club developed and delivered a bespoke behavioural intervention focussed on the promotion of healthy lifestyles, based on the assessment of local needs. To achieve this end, project staff formed local steering groups that included local men, delivery agents and strategic partners involved in developing Joint Strategic Needs Assessments and Local Area Agreements.

PLH was delivered free of charge by community coaching staff, Health Trainers and allied health professionals employed by participating clubs. All interventions – as a minimum requirement – ran one PLH session each week lasting approximately 90 min. Each 90-min session typically incorporated practical physical activity (commonly football, cricket, volleyball, badminton, cycling or circuit training), combined with *lifestyle advice* classes/seminars (advocating the benefits of a healthy lifestyle). Within this time frame, approximately one hour was set aside for 'doing' physical activity; and the remaining time was used to deliver *lifestyle advice*. The weighting and content of classroom and physical activity sessions changed over the intervention period. For example, in some interventions, as participants increased their fitness, the classroom element became shorter, focusing on reviewing earlier sessions to check understanding and self-monitoring individual goals. In other interventions, topics for classroom sessions and modes of activity altered in line with participant requests and requirements. Notwithstanding programme content, delivery across the clubs was underpinned by a strong sense of informality and a concern for engagement and enjoyment. Interventions took place between October 2009 and July 2012.

Study population

The data *corpus* comprised 4020 men. Data were excluded from the current analysis where (i) participants only engaged one-off match-day-type events ($n = 1056$), with no possibility of follow-up, or (ii) if there was missing data for any lifestyle risk factors at pre- or post-intervention ($n = 1297$). The resulting data set comprised 1667 (56%) men aged 18–75 years.

Data collection: demographics, lifestyle risk factors and covariates

Prior to data collection, ethical approval was obtained from the research ethics committee at Leeds Beckett University. Further, all procedures and instrumentation were piloted and refined prior to use.[27] Intervention staff collected pre-intervention measures at first point of contact, typically at pre-activity assessments and inductions along with informed consent. Data were then captured again at a 12-week follow-up. The structured questionnaire assessed socio-demographics (age, ethnicity, employment status) along with lifestyle risk factors (diet, activity, smoking and alcohol) and covariates (stress-related health and social support).

Although objective measurement of these lifestyle risk factors is desirable in many circumstances, a number of self-report measures are valid, reliable and often the most practical in real-world community evaluations.[28] Further, they can be sufficiently sensitive to detect change in behaviour.[29] Moreover, self-report remains an integral and accessible methodology for widespread public health surveillance. For example, the majority of data supporting a link between habitual physical activity and chronic disease stem from self-report.[30] Selecting the 'correct' measurement tool/method is not simply about having the most accurate – objective – measure, but more about being aware of the underlying mechanisms that should guide selection. Even objective measures have their own set of limitations and sources of measurement error.[31] Nevertheless, self-report is often rebuked even when it is the most appropriate and logical method of data capture.

Four lifestyle risk factors were assessed in this study using valid and reliable measures. In line with current recommendations[32] and to assess physical activity, participants were asked how many days during the last week they accumulated ≥ 30 min of at least moderate intensity physical activity.[33] Not meeting this criterion was classed as a lifestyle risk factor. Diet was assessed by summing all the portions of pulses, salads, vegetables, fruit juices and fresh, canned and dried fruit eaten on an 'average' day. Consumption of less than five daily portions was considered a lifestyle risk factor.[34] Alcohol risk was assessed using UK Health guidelines,[35] questions focussed on how many units of alcohol participants consumed weekly; consumption of ≥ 21 units weekly was considered excessive, therefore qualifying as a risk factor. Participants reporting the current use of tobacco were classed as smokers, and therefore possessed this risk factor.[36] To assess stress-related health, participants were asked,[37] 'In the last month, have you felt that you were under so much stress that your health was likely to suffer'? Responses were dichotomized in to (i) 'never' and (ii) 'yes'. Social support networks were assessed by asking participants 'Do you have people you can rely on in times of trouble'? Responses were dichotomized in to (i) 'never' and (ii) 'yes'.

Statistical analyses

Descriptive characteristics of the population are described for demographics and covariates. A multiple lifestyle risk factor index ranging from 0 (no risk factors) to 4 (all four risk factors) was developed, along with a dichotomized index of low risk (no, one and two risk factors) and high risk (three and four risk factors). For prevalence, the number and percentage of each individual lifestyle risk factor and each possible combination is reported.

Chi-square tests assessed demographic variations. A multinomial logistic regression model estimated the probability that – at recruitment – a participant had lifestyle risk factors compared to a reference group of '0'. Wilcoxon signed-rank tests assessed differences in individual and total lifestyle risk factors, and between participants presenting high and low lifestyle risk from pre- to post-intervention. Pearson's correlation coefficient effect sizes were calculated to standardize the measure of the effect observed $(r = z/\sqrt{N})$.[38] For all inferential tests, a p value of <0.05 was taken to be statistically significant. Analyses were conducted using SPSS for windows version 19.0.

Results

Table 1 shows the baseline characteristics of participants; they were predominantly aged 18–34 years (51.6%, $n = 865$), from a white British background (71.6%, $n = 1181$) and in employment (57.6%, $n = 932$). A significantly larger proportion of excluded participants were aged 18–34 years $(\chi^2[1] = 30.23, p < 0.001)$, from Black and minority ethnic backgrounds $(\chi^2[1] = 7.02, p < 0.05)$, and currently in employment $(\chi^2[1] = 13.52, p < 0.001)$.

Table 1. Characteristics of the study population pre-intervention.

		% of participants (n)
Socio-demographics		
Age ($n = 1656$)	18–24	26.1% (433)
	25–34	25.5% (423)
	35–44	25.6% (424)
	45–54	15.5% (256)
	55–64	5.4% (90)
	≥65	1.8% (30)
Ethnicity ($n = 1649$)	White British	71.6% (1181)
	Black and minority ethnic	28.4% (468)
Employment status ($n = 1619$)	Employed	57.6% (932)
	Unemployed	42.4% (687)
Lifestyle risk factors		
Smoking($n = 1667$)	Current smoker	31.3% (522)
Excessive drinking ($n = 1667$)	≥21 units of alcohol/week	29.7% (495)
Lack of fruit/vegetables ($n = 1667$)	<5 portions/day	88.1% (1468)
Lack of physical activity ($n = 1667$)	<5× 300 min sessions/week	84.9% (1416)
Number of risk factors ($n = 1667$)	4	9.7% (162)
	3	31.7% (529)
	2	44.2% (737)
	1	11.5% (192)
	0	2.8% (47)
Covariates		
Health suffered due to stress ($n = 1563$)	Never	55.2% (862)
	Yes	44.8% (701)
Social support in times of trouble	Never	39.7% (624)
($n = 1573$)		
	Yes	60.3% (949)

Note: The disparity in sample size for selected variables was due to participants not completing all sections of the data capture.

Regarding adherence to health-enhancing behavioural recommendations at baseline, around 85% ($n = 1468$) of the men under-exercised, 88% ($n = 1416$) did not eat enough fruit and vegetables daily, 31% ($n = 522$) smoked and 30% ($n = 495$) drank excessively. Few (3%, $n = 47$) presented no lifestyle risk factors, 11% ($n = 192$) had one and 42% ($n = 737$) had two lifestyle risk factors. Over 32% ($n = 529$) combined three lifestyle risk factors and around 10% ($n = 162$) had all four. More than 55% ($n = 862$) of the men reported that their health had suffered due to stress in the last month, and around 40% ($n = 624$) reported not having social support networks to rely on in times of trouble.

Table 2 shows a multinomial multilevel logistic regression model, with the number of baseline lifestyle risk factors as the dependent variable. Men aged ≥ 35 years were 55% less likely to display all four risk factors (Odds Ratio [OR]: 0.45, 95% Confidence Interval [CI]: 0.23–0.88) compared to those aged 18–34 years, and the likelihood of presenting all four risk factors was reduced by 83% among men who thought that their health had not suffered in the last month due to stress (OR: 0.17, 95% CI: 0.08–0.36) compared to men reporting that it had. Unemployed men were three and a half times more likely to present multiple lifestyle risk factors compared to employed men (OR: 3.64, 95% CI: 1.78–7.51). Further, men who reported having no social support networks to rely on in times of trouble had the greatest odds for reporting all four lifestyle risk factors (OR: 5.10, 95% CI: 2.44–10.50). Assessments of post-intervention change indicated no significant differences in the profiles between those men that changed compared to those that did not, indicating equivalent responsiveness to the intervention.

Table 3 shows the prevalence of all 16 possible combinations of lifestyle risk factors at pre- and post-intervention. At pre-intervention, the four most common risk factor combinations included under exercising and poor diet (77%). This pattern remained at post-intervention (74%). The number of lifestyle risk factors reported significantly reduced from pre- to post-intervention ($z = -7.488$, $p < 0.001$, $r = -0.13$). Further, there was a significant reduction in the number of participants ($n = 51$) presenting a high lifestyle risk at post-intervention ($z = -6.326$, $p < 0.001$, $r = -0.11$).

Individually, at post-intervention, there were statistically significant improvements in physical activity ($z = -12.446$ $p < 0.001$, $r = -0.22$), over 15% ($n = 254$) of men increased their activity, while 2.9% ($n = 50$) were now meeting current recommendations. Fruit and vegetable consumption also significantly improved ($z = -11.652$ $p < 0.001$, $r = -0.20$), more than 13% ($n = 222$) of men increased their intake, 1.9% ($n = 33$) went on to meet current recommendations. Alcohol intake was significantly reduced ($z = -9.419$ $p < 0.001$, $r = -0.16$), around 10% ($n = 170$) reduced their weekly intake with over 2.7% ($n = 45$) reducing it to meet current guidelines. Finally, the incidence of smoking was significantly reduced ($z = -2.921$ $p < 0.001$, $r = -0.05$), 1.4% ($n = 23$) of men stopped smoking.

Discussion

This study investigated the most influential predictors of simultaneous lifestyle risk factors in men and identified the effects of a 12-week men's health promotion intervention delivered in and by English Premier League football clubs. To our knowledge, this is the first study of its type to investigate these issues with this group. Results highlight an elevated risk for multiple combinations of lifestyle risk factors

Table 2. Odds ratios and 95% confidence intervals for predictors of lifestyle risk factors pre-intervention.

	One lifestyle risk factor			Two lifestyle risk factors			Three lifestyle risk factors			Four lifestyle risk factors		
	OR	95% CI		OR	95% CI		OR	95% CI		OR	95% CI	
Age												
(18–34)												
35+	0.93	0.49–1.79	n.s.	0.69	0.97–1.26	n.s.	0.77	0.42–1.41	n.s.	0.45	0.23–0.88	*
Employment												
(Employed)												
Unemployed	1.66	0.82–3.37	n.s.	1.60	0.82–3.10	n.s.	2.01	1.11–4.10	*	3.64	1.78–7.51	***
Ethnicity												
(White British)												
BME	1.24	0.51–2.30	n.s.	2.75	1.22–6.24	*	1.33	0.58–3.10	n.s.	0.87	0.35–2.19	n.s.
Suffered from stress												
(Yes)												
Never	0.99	0.50–1.98	n.s.	0.49	0.26–9.32	*	0.34	0.18–0.64	**	0.17	0.08–0.36	***
Social support												
(Yes)												
Never	0.78	0.40–1.61	n.s	2.10	1.10–3.90	*	2.20	1.15–4.20	*	5.10	2.44–10.50	***

Note: n.s. = non-significant; the reference group of predictor variables are given in parentheses, BME = Black and minority ethnic.
*$p < 0.05$; **$p < 0.01$; ***$p < 0.001$.

Table 3. Descriptive combination pattern for lifestyle risk factors.

Number of risk factors	Identified lifestyle risk factors				Prevalence	
	Poor diet	Physically inactive	Current smoker	Excessive alcohol	Pre % (n)	Post % (n)
4	✔	✔	✔	✔	9.7 (162)	9.2 (154)
3	✔	✔	✔	×	15.8 (263)	15.1 (252)
	✔	✔	×	✔	14.3 (238)	12.5 (209)
	✔	×	✔	✔	1.4 (24)	1.3 (22)
	×	✔	✔	✔	0.2 (4)	0.2 (3)
					31.7 (529)	29.1 (486)
2	✔	✔	×	×	37.3 (621)	38.0 (633)
	✔	×	✔	×	2.0 (33)	2.2 (37)
	✔	×	×	✔	2.5 (41)	2.6 (44)
	×	✔	✔	×	1.3 (22)	1.4 (23)
	×	✔	×	✔	1.1 (18)	1.0 (16)
	×	×	✔	✔	0.1 (2)	0.1 (1)
					44.2 (737)	45.2 (754)
1	✔	×	×	×	5.2 (86)	5.6 (93)
	×	✔	×	×	5.3 (88)	5.4 (90)
	×	×	✔	×	0.7 (12)	0.9 (15)
	×	×	×	✔	0.4 (6)	0.5 (8)
					11.5 (192)	12.4 (206)
0	×	×	×	×	2.8 (47)	4.0 (67)

Note: ✔ = Lifestyle risk factor present, × = Lifestyle risk factor absent, Pre = Lifestyle risk factor combination pre-intervention, Post = Lifestyle risk factor combination post-intervention. The underlined values are subtotals for the % of participants reporting 1, 2 and 3 lifestyle risk factors.

at pre-intervention in those men who were unemployed, under stress and with poor social support networks. This attests to effective recruitment. The 12-week intervention helped to positively alter individual, and combinations of the most potent risk factors for non-communicable disease in men typically viewed as being unresponsive to health-focused interventions and hard-to-connect with.

Our finding that the strongest predictor of multiple concurrent lifestyle risk involves poor social support networks is important and consistent with other data.[39] In their own right, pre-existing social support and social networks established through sporting associations have the potential to minimize attrition and regression towards unhealthy practices.[40] PLH provided access to these networks for many of the recruits who were socially isolated when the programme began; we suggest that the association with football provided an approach that was also socially acceptable and desirable to participants. Further, the football context was comfortable, familiar, inclusive, and –as the intervention outcomes show – assisted men to overcome many barriers to better health. Therefore, health interventions aimed at marginalized groups should incorporate components designed to improve social support and social networks.

At recruitment, unhealthy behaviours were common, which confirms effective targeting and recruitment. Physical inactivity and poor diet was the most prevalent combination among men presenting three and four lifestyle risk factors, suggesting a connection to non-adherence with tobacco and alcohol recommendations. Given that PLH was centred on physical activity, the reductions witnessed in other, seemingly unrelated risk factors, suggest that increased physical activity may have the potential to catalyse positive changes in other lifestyle behaviours. This is important for establishing which lifestyle behaviours are the most effective at eliciting change in other behaviours and therefore, which to target first. However, previous UK evidence[41] has also shown that the most active men are also more likely to smoke and over-consume alcohol. Therefore, the links between these behaviours – and their modification – need to be assessed carefully.

Debates surrounding combinations vs. sequential methods of lifestyle behaviour change amplify the need to gauge the size of the effect in combination, as well as individually. Outcomes from PLH indicated a small, yet significant effect for reductions in combinations with lifestyle risk factors over 12 weeks. Previous studies involving men in football settings have also found significant reductions in risk factors over a similar time period,[42] but delivered to far fewer men than in PLH. This notwithstanding, the results are encouraging especially given the well-documented difficulties that many practitioners experience when attempting to engage this group with health promotion.[43] Stronger research designs are needed to provide the evidence to consider health interventions in football – or indeed sporting contexts – as a major public breakthrough.

Regarding individual behaviours, the largest intervention effect was found for increased physical activity. Yet, only a small number of insufficiently active participants improved to meet current recommendations. The high baseline incidence of inactivity – over 50% of men undertook ≤ 2 sessions of physical activity per week at pre-intervention – and/or the dichotomized risk factor variables may account for this modest scale of effect. Therefore, accumulation of one or two additional sessions may be seen as an accomplishment for some men. For others, maintaining current activity – even if low – represents a considerable achievement within the intervention.

Unhealthy groups can find it particularly challenging to sustain behaviour change. The divergent patterns of lifestyle risk factors shown in the current study – at baseline and follow-up – provide challenges and opportunities for public health. Behaviour change is reinforced by tangible short-term effects, like feeling fitter, compared to longer term effects like reducing risk for non-communicable disease.[44] Consequently, interventions where the short-term benefits – including better physical performance – represent lifestyle change in their own right are more likely to be sustained, which contributes to their effectiveness. While this study shows that an initial intervention period can initiate change and stabilize problematic behaviours, establishing more permanent change is more challenging. The effectiveness of population-based multiple behaviour interventions need to be established for both short-term change and longer term maintenance of multiple acquired behaviours.[45]

Compared to men demonstrating no change, the current data show no significant differences in baseline profiles among men who improved their risk factor status. Pre-intervention, the majority of participants who achieved positive lifestyle change harboured poor social support networks and thought that their health had suffered due to stress pre-intervention. These were the most influential predictors of multiple lifestyle risk, yet in the current study, they were not impediments to change. This highlights the capacity of sporting settings to tackle the key determinants of healthy lifestyles in those men with the most problematic health profiles and revises the notion of these men being resistant to change.

Outcomes from this study reflect a number of limitations, including the lack of a control condition and the non-random selection of participants. Further, basing lifestyle risk factors on UK health recommendations may make it difficult to generalize the findings to different settings and populations. The data are also based on self-report which may be subject to participant bias and socially desirable responses; therefore, an unknown level of misclassification may have occurred. The common practice of dichotomizing health behaviour variables may have implications for the findings,[46] while the effects may have been attributable to factors other than the intervention. With these thoughts in mind, future studies should seek to assess outcomes from a longitudinal perspective using more rigorous experimental designs and objective measures of lifestyle risk factors where possible.

The most economically disadvantaged individuals and those with the lowest education often benefit least from health interventions, leading to widening inequalities and avoidable pressure on health services.[47] Achieved at a population level, even the modest scale of the positive improvements in combinations of lifestyle behaviours reported through this intervention, can have immense benefits for health services. Yet, unresolved, these issues increase the healthcare burden and the incidence of non-communicable disease in later life. This study found younger, unemployed men with poor social networks and higher levels of stress at an increased likelihood of presenting multiple lifestyle risk factors. Further, a 12-week health promotion intervention delivered in and by professional football clubs had a positive effect on reducing risk factors and improving lifestyles. These outcomes show that men are not universally resistant to lifestyle change, and they can respond positively to behaviourally-focused interventions if they are delivered in places and settings that are local and familiar, yet prestigious.

Acknowlededgements

The authors wish to thank all the individuals and agencies who partnered PLH, including the Football Pools, the FA Premier League, the participants and staff in the 16 EPL clubs, their local partners, and people in the authors' organizations who supported this work.

Disclosure statement

No potential conflict of interest was reported by the authors.

Funding

The Programme was supported by the FA Premier League (the commissioners) with funding provided by the Football Pools (the sponsors).

Notes

1. European Commission, *The State of Men's Health in Europe*.
2. Sinclair and Alexander, 'Outreach to Involve the Hard-to-reach'.
3. Priest et al., *Interventions Implemented through Sporting Organisations*.
4. White et al., 'Engaging Men in Health Interventions'.
5. Laaksonen, Prattala, and Lahelma, 'Determinants of Unhealthy Lifestyle Behaviours'; Pronk et al., 'Optimal Lifestyles'; Shankar, McMunn, and Steptoe, 'Socioeconomic Status and Health'.
6. White et al., 'Innovative Approaches for Improving Men's Health'.
7. Pringle and Sayers, 'Community Based Mental Health with Football'.
8. Turk et al., 'Randomised Trials of Weight Loss in Men'.

9. Brady et al., 'Men's Health through Football in Scotland'.
10. McGale, McArdle, and Gaffney, 'Effectiveness of CBT for Young Men'.
11. Darongkamas, Scott, and Taylor, 'Men's Mental Health, the Effect of Playing Football'.
12. White et al., 'Social Relationships in Men'.
13. Berkman et al., 'Social Integration and Health'.
14. White et al., 'Engaging Men in Health Interventions'.
15. Cohen, 'Social Relationships and Health'.
16. Holt-Lunstad, Smith, and Layton, 'Relationships and Mortality'.
17. Poortinga, 'Lifestyle Risk Factor Clustering'; World Health Organization, *Non-communicable Disease*.
18. Department of Health, *NHS Future Forum*.
19. Ford, Greenlund, and Hong, 'Cardiovascular Health and Mortality'.
20. Buck and Frosini, 'Unhealthy Behaviour Clustering'.
21. Chiolero et al., 'Clustering of Risk'; Poortinga, 'Lifestyle Risk Factor Clustering'; Schuit et al., 'Lifestyle Risk in Adults'.
22. Jackson, 'Behaviour Change in Health Education'.
23. Poortinga, 'Lifestyle Risk Factor Clustering'; Schuit, 'Prevalence of LRFs in Adults'.
24. Bassuk and Manson, 'Lifestyle and Disease Link'.
25. Khaw et al., 'Health Behaviours and Mortality'.
26. Pringle et al., 'Demographic and Health Profiles of Men Engaging PLH'.
27. South and Tilford, 'Research and Evaluation – Influences on Activity'.
28. Buck and Frosini, 'Unhealthy Behaviour Clustering'; Chiolero et al., 'Clustering of Risk'; Dodd et al., 'Lifestyle Risk in Students'; Fine et al., 'Multiple Chronic Disease Risk Factors'; Poortinga, 'Lifestyle Risk Factor Clustering'; Pringle et al., 'Cost Effectiveness of Community Activity Interventions'; Schuit et al., 'Lifestyle Risk in Adults'.
29. Khaw et al., 'Health Behaviours and Mortality in Men and Women'.
30. Haskell, 'Physical Activity by Self-report'.
31. Sternfeld and Goldman-Rosas, 'Appropriate Measures of Self-report'.
32. Department of Health, *Start Active Stay Active*.
33. Marcus and Forsyth, *Motivating People to Become Active*.
34. NICE, *Assessment of Overweight and Obesity*.
35. Department of Health, *Alcohol Guidelines*.
36. Vaananen et al., 'Smoking Assessment'.
37. American Psychological Association, *Stress Related Health*.
38. Rosenthal, *Statistical Procedures for Social Research*.
39. Holt-Lunstad, Smith, and Layton, 'Relationships and Mortality'.
40. White et al., 'Engaging Men in Health Interventions'.
41. Poortinga, 'Lifestyle Risk Factor Clustering'; Schuit et al., 'Lifestyle Risk in Adults'.
42. Brady et al., 'Men's Health through Football in Scotland'.
43. Turk et al., 'Randomised Trials of Weight Loss in Men'.
44. Jackson, 'Behaviour Change in Health Education'.
45. Berrigan et al., 'Patterns of Health Behaviour'.
46. MacCallum et al., 'Dichotomizing Quantitative Variables'.
47. Chiolero et al., 'Clustering of Risk'; Poortinga, 'Lifestyle Risk Factor Clustering'; Schuit et al., 'Lifestyle Risk in Adults'.

References

American Psychological Association. *Stress in America: Our Health at Risk*. Washington, DC: American Psychological Association, 2012.

Bassuk, S., and J. Manson. 'Lifestyle and Risk of Cardiovascular Disease and Type 2 Diabetes in Women: A Review of the Epidemiologic Evidence'. *American Journal of Lifestyle Medicine* 2 (2008): 191–213.

Berkman, L., T. Glass, I. Brissette, and T. Seeman. 'From Social Integration to Health: Durkheim in the New Millennium'. *Social Science and Medicine* 51 (2000): 843–57.

Berrigan, D., K. Dodd, R. Troiano, S. Krebs-Smith, and R. Barbash. 'Patterns of Health Behavior in U.S. Adults'. *Preventive Medicine* 36 (2003): 615–23.

Brady, A., C. Perry, D. Murdoch, and G. McKay. 'Sustained Benefits of a Health Project for Middle Aged Football Supporters, at Glasgow Celtic and Rangers Football Clubs'. *European Heart Journal* 24 (2010): 2696–8.

Buck, D., and F. Frosini. *Clustering of Unhealthy Behaviours over Time: Implications for Policy and Practice.* Ed. T.K. Fund. London: The Kings Fund, 2010.

Chiolero, A., V. Wietlisbach, C. Ruffieux, F. Paccaud, and J. Cornuz. 'Clustering of Risk Behaviors with Cigarette Consumption: A Population-based Survey'. *Preventive Medicine* 42 (2006): 348–53.

Cohen, S. 'Social Relationships and Health'. *American Psychologist* 59 (2004): 676–84.

Darongkamas, J., H. Scott, and E. Taylor. 'Kick-starting Men's Mental Health: An Evaluation of the Effect of Playing Football on Mental Health Service Users' Well-being'. *International Journal of Mental Health Promotion* 13 (2011): 14–21.

Department of Health. *How Much is Too Much? Drinking and You.* London: Department of Health, 2007.

Department of Health. *Start Active, Stay Active: A Report on Physical Activity for Health from the Four Home Countries. Chief Medical Officer.* London: Department of Health, 2011.

Department of Health. *Government Response to NHS Future Forum's Second Report.* London: Department of Health, 2012. www.dh.gov.uk/en/Publicationsandstatistics/Publications/PublicationsPolicyAndGuidance?DH_132075 (accessed August 12, 2014).

Dodd, L., Y. Al-Nakeeb, A. Nevill, and M. Forshaw. 'Lifestyle Risk Factors of Students: A Cluster Analytical Approach'. *Preventive Medicine* 51 (2010): 73–7.

European Commission. *The State of Men's Health in Europe Report.* European Commission, 2011. http://ec.europa.eu/health/population_groups/docs/men_health_report_en.pdf (accessed July 9, 2014).

Fine, L., S. Philogene, R. Gramling, E. Coups, and S. Sinha. 'Prevalence of Multiple Chronic Disease Risk Factors: 2001 National Health Interview Survey'. *American Journal of Preventive Medicine* 27 (2004): 18–24.

Ford, E., K. Greenlund, and Y. Hong. 'Ideal Cardiovascular Health and Mortality from All Causes and Diseases of the Circulatory System among Adults in the United States'. *Circulation* 125 (2012): 987–95.

Haskell, W. 'Physical Activity by Self-report: A Brief History and Future Issues'. *Journal of Physical Activity and Health* 9 (2012): S5–S10.

Holt-Lunstad, J., T. Smith, and J. Layton. 'Social Relationships and Mortality Risk: A Meta-analytic Review'. *PLoS Medicine* 7 (2010): e1000316.

Jackson, C. 'Behavioral Science Theory and Principles for Practice in Health Education'. *Health Education Research* 12 (1997): 143–50.

Khaw, K., N. Wareham, S. Bingham, A. Welch, R. Luben, and N. Day. 'Combined Impact of Health Behaviours and Mortality in Men and Women: The EPIC-Norfolk Prospective Population Study'. *PLoS Medicine* 5 (2008): 39–47.

Laaksonen, M., R. Prattala, and E. Lahelma. 'Sociodemographic Determinants of Multiple Unhealthy Behaviours'. *Scandinavian Journal of Public Health* 31 (2003): 37–43.

MacCallum, R., S. Zhang, K. Preacher, and D. Rucker. 'On the Practice of Dichotomization of Quantitative Variables'. *Psychological Methods* 7 (2002): 19–40.

Marcus, B., and L. Forsyth. *Motivating People to Become Physically Active.* 2nd ed. Champaign, IL, Human Kinetics, 2009.

McGale, N., S. McArdle, and P. Gaffney. 'Exploring the Effectiveness of an Integrated Exercise/CBT Intervention for Young Men's Mental Health'. *British Journal of Health Psychology* 16 (2011): 457–71.

National Institute of Health and Clinical Excellence. *Guidance on the Prevention, Identification, Assessment and Management of Overweight and Obesity in Adults and Children.* London: National Institute of Health and Clinical Excellence, 2006.

Poortinga, W. 'The Prevalence and Clustering of Four Major Lifestyle Risk Factors in an English Adult Population'. *Preventive Medicine* 44 (2007): 124–8.

Priest, N., R. Armstrong, J. Doyle, and E. Waters. 'Interventions Implemented Through Sporting Organisations for Increasing Participation in Sport', *Cochrane Database of Systematic Reviews*, no. 3 (2008). Article ID: CD004812. DOI: 10.1002/14651858. CD004812.pub3.

Pringle, A., C. Cooke, N. Gilson, K. Marsh, and J. McKenna. 'Cost-effectiveness of Interventions to Improve Moderate Physical Activity: A Study in Nine UK Sites'. *Health Education Journal* 69 (2010): 211–24.

Pringle, A., and P. Sayers. 'It's a Goal!: Basing a Community Psychiatric Nursing Service in a Local Football Stadium'. *The Journal of the Royal Society for the Promotion of Health* 124 (2006): 234–8.

Pringle, A., S. Zwolinsky, A. Smith, S. Robertson, J. McKenna, and A. White. 'The Pre-adoption Demographic and Health Profiles of Men Participating in a Programme of Men's Health Delivered in English Premier League Football Clubs'. *Public Health* 125 (2011): 411–6.

Pronk, N., M. Lowry, T. Kottke, E. Austin, J. Gallagher, and A. Katz. 'The Association between Optimal Lifestyle Adherence and Short-term Incidence of Chronic Conditions among Employees'. *Population Health Management* 13 (2010): 289–95.

Rosenthal, R. *Meta-analytic Procedures for Social Research*. 2nd ed. Newbury Park, CA: Sage, 1991.

Schuit, A., A. van Loon, M. Tijhuis, and M. Ocké. 'Clustering of Lifestyle Risk Factors in a General Adult Population'. *Preventive Medicine* 35 (2002): 219–24.

Shankar, A., A. McMunn, and A. Steptoe. 'Health-related Behaviors in Older Adults'. *American Journal of Preventive Medicine* 38 (2010): 39–46.

Sinclair, A., and H. Alexander. 'Using Outreach to Involve the Hard-to-reach in a Health Check: What Difference Does It Make?' *Public Health* 126 (2012): 87–95.

South, J., and S. Tilford. 'Perceptions of Research and Evaluation in Health Promotion Practice and Influences on Activity'. *Health Education Research* 15 (2000): 729–41.

Sternfeld, B., and L. Goldman-Rosas. 'A Systematic Approach to Selecting an Appropriate Measure of Self-reported Physical Activity or Sedentary Behaviour'. *Journal of Physical Activity and Health* 9 (2012): S19–28.

Turk, M., K. Yang, M. Hravnak, S. Sereika, L. Ewing, and L. Burke. 'Randomized Clinical Trials of Weight Loss Maintenance'. *The Journal of Cardiovascular Nursing* 24 (2009): 58–80.

Vaananen, A., A. Kouvonen, M. Kivimaki, T. Oksanen, M. Elovainio, M. Virtanen, and J. Pentti. 'Workplace Social Capital and Co-occurrence of Lifestyle Risk Factors: The Finnish Public Sector Study'. *Occupational and Environmental Medicine* 66 (2009): 432–7.

Vartiainen, E., T. Seppala, and P. Puska. 'Validation of Self-reported Smoking by Serum Cotinine Measurement in a Community-based Study'. *Journal of Epidemiology and Community Health* 56 (2002): 167–70.

White, A., M. McKee, N. Richardson, R. Visser, S. Madsen, B. Sousa, and P. Makara. 'Europe's Men Need Their Own Health Strategy'. *British Medical Journal* (2011): 343. doi:10.1136/bmj.d7397.

World Health Organization. *Scaling up Action against Non-communicable Diseases: How Much will It Cost?* Geneva: World Health Organization, 2011.

Effectiveness of a community football programme on improving physiological markers of health in a hard-to-reach male population: the role of exercise intensity

Andrew Thomas Hulton[a], David Flower[b], Rebecca Murphy[a], Dave Richardson[a], Barry Drust[a] and Kathryn Curran[c]

[a]The Football Exchange, Research Institute for Sport and Exercise Sciences, Liverpool John Moores University, Liverpool, UK; [b]Everton Football Club, Liverpool, UK; [c]Carnegie Faculty, Centre for Active Lifestyles, Institute for Sport, Physical Activity and Leisure, Leeds Beckett University, Leeds, UK

The present study evaluated the effectiveness of participation in recreational football during a community health programme, on physiological markers of health within a hard to reach population. Nine men (Age: 33 ± 9 years, Mass: 75.4 ± 13.7 kg, Height: 1.74 ± 0.07 m and Body Fat: $19 \pm 2\%$) were recruited to participate in the study in collaboration with an English Premier League Football Club. Participants completed the 12-week football-based programme which included two coached football sessions each week. Physiological tests for blood pressure, resting heart rate, cholesterol and an anthropometrical test for body composition were completed at three time points during the study (Weeks – 1, 6 and 12) in an attempt to evaluate the impact of the intervention on health. During each training session, measurements of intensity ($\%HR_{max}$, identified from the yoyo intermittent level 1 test), duration and rating of perceived exertion were made. The 12-week programme (mean HR_{max} throughout programme = $75 \pm 4\%$ beats min^{-1}; mean RPE throughout programme = 6 ± 1) elicited few changes in physiological markers of health with the only significant change been a decrease in resting heart rate from weeks 6 to 12 (87 ± 22 beats min^{-1} at week-6, to 72 ± 17 beats min^{-1}; $p < 0.05$). These data would suggest that the current community football-related health project was not effective in improving physiological markers of health, but was able to maintain their level of health. A lack of improvement may be due to the low intensity of sessions and a lack of coach education for the promotion of sessions that aim to improve health.

Introduction

The uptake of traditional health services (General Practices) by men is a cause for concern amongst public health professionals in the UK.[1] Individuals from hard-to-reach (HTR) populations experience difficulty engaging in physical activity for a sustained period of time.[2] Hard-to-reach populations are those who are difficult to access due to a specific factor that characterizes its members (homeless people, prostitutes, drug addicts), which results in marginalization and restricted access to appropriate health care due to social barriers created by ignorance, prejudice and discrimination[3] from the general population. Targeting health intervention is therefore an important factor in engaging HTR male populations who may be predisposed to cardiovascular health concerns.[4]

Interventions that use popular sports such as football as the exercise stimulus have been developed as a way to engage with HTR populations. Football may have a great potential to act as a health promotion tool as a consequence of its ability to improve the motivational and social factors associated with its participation when compared to more traditional types of exercise interventions such as continuous moderate intensity running.[5] In order to remove the barriers for male participation, it has been suggested[6] that sports groups may serve as the most appropriate community setting for these populations, as traditional health care advice is typically dominated by female friendly practises which make male populations regard themselves as intruders.[7] Until recently, few studies have investigated the health effects of football training, small sided game (SSG) play and match play.[8] These investigations, typically conducted over 12 weeks with two–three 60 min sessions per week, have shown positive health benefits linked to football participation such as muscular hypertrophy and increases in strength,[9] a decrease in blood pressure,[10] a decrease in total fat mass[11] as well as an increase in $\dot{V}0_{2max}$.[12] Therefore, there may be a potential for football to remove the social barriers commonly perceived by the HTR population, and allow these interventions to provide the many health benefits observed within the literature.

Research into the health effects of recreational football[13] to date has typically employed well-controlled experimental designs that predominately utilize carefully prescribed football-related activities. Furthermore, participants within these investigations are typically healthy and untrained who volunteer for the research. Such programmes are also typified by high levels of compliance to study requirements and regular attendance at sessions throughout the training programme. Golay et al. suggested[14] that 'real-life' participation in such programmes or trials do not necessarily reflect study cohorts and can be influenced from factors outside the realm of the programme or trial. The framework employed within much of the previous literature may therefore not reflect the reality of provision within a typical community-based programme that uses skills coaches to deliver football sessions as a vehicle for health promotion. Such programmes, where the structure of training activities and the level of participant commitment may be more varied, may have the potential to reduce the effectiveness of football-based interventions. These concerns could be further amplified by participants from HTR populations who decline formal treatment, lack motivation and lead unconventional lifestyles.

The present study aimed to evaluate the effectiveness of regular participation in recreational football, as part of a Football in the Community (FitC) health programme, on markers of health within a hard-to-reach population.

Materials and methods

Experimental design

All participants were involved in a 12-week football-coached intervention programme. Two football sessions lasting 120 min in duration were completed each week as the exercise stimulus, with HR continually monitored to measure exercise intensity, following the measurement of HR_{max} (described below). To evaluate the health impact of the intervention, health-related physiological testing was completed at three time points during the study (Weeks – 1, 6 and 12).This included body composition, blood pressure and cholesterol. Participants were familiarized with the training programme, testing procedures and gave their written informed consent to participate in the study and provide all additional measurements in accordance with the ethical clearance provided by the universities' ethics committee prior to the study completion.

Participants

Nine men (Age: 33 ± 9 years, Mass: 75.4 ± 13.7 kg, Height: 1.74 ± 0.07 m and Body Fat: $19 \pm 2\%$) were recruited to participate in the study from a men's homeless shelter and a drug addiction service, who were already in partnership with the FitC health programme at an English Premier League Football Club. Participants were recruited using a variety of mechanisms including face-to-face engagement, phone calls, referrals from service staff and word of mouth. The majority of the participants were smokers, had a history of drug use (though were recovering and had not taken drugs for at least 6 months) and did not regularly participate in any form of structured physical exercise. Participants were deemed healthy and able to participate following responses given to standardized health questions. These included previous and current medical information around cardiorespiratory, bone and joint health.

In total, 20 participants signed up to the programme; however, 11 dropped out during the course of the study leaving the final sample to comprise nine individuals. Reasons for participant drop out included: depression and mental health issues (causing a lack of engagement), lack of motivation to attend sessions and trouble with local authorities. The average percentage of attendance of participants to training sessions throughout the programme was $84 \pm 7\%$. Reasons for non-attendance during the programme included: illness, injury, family issues and situational issues, such as lack of money to travel to the training venue and obligatory appointments with social workers.

Training intervention

Outdoor training was completed two times per week for 12 weeks on a 20 m by 30 m artificial pitch. Each training session was scheduled for 120 min. Football sessions were conducted by a qualified FitC coach and generally followed a similar format. Typically, this involved a standardised 10-min warm-up composed of gentle jogging, dynamic, football-related movements (e.g. side-steps, skipping, jumping and lunges), sprinting and dynamic and static stretching. Twenty to thirty min of technical practice (defined as: Individual or group practice covering technical elements under no pressure) was performed, followed by ~20–30 min of skills practice (defined as: Individual or group practice covering technical elements under opposed pressure), or possession games (defined as: Practice in which ball retention, rather than scoring a goal is the primary objective).[15] The sessions were concluded with ~30–40 min of SSG (6v6, 5v5 or 4v4). Sessions differed from this format in weeks 1, 6 and 12 when physical fitness testing was completed during the first session of the week.

HR telemetry was continuously monitored throughout football sessions and was recorded every 5 s using HR monitors (Polar Team System, Polar, Kempele, Finland). The mean HR of each individual training activity (i.e. warm up, technical practice, skills/possession practice and SSG) was determined and used for analysis. The mean HR collected throughout the entire session provided an indication of the overall session intensity. Participant's maximal HR (HR_{max}) was determined from the HR peak recorded during the Yo-Yo Intermittent Endurance Level 1(Yo-Yo IE1) test. This enabled the collected HR data to also be expressed as a percentage of the individuals HR_{max}. Rating of perceived exertion (RPE) was collected at the end of each session and determined using Borg's CR10-scale.[16] Training load (RPE_{load}) was determined by multiplying the training duration (minutes) by the session RPE, as previously described.[17] This RPE-based method of training load quantification has been shown to be a good indicator of internal training load in football.[18]

Testing procedures and measurements

Testing was completed three times during the study (Weeks 1, 6 and 12), with participant's attending the laboratory for health screening. All testing procedures were explained and demonstrated to participants prior to the completion of the assessment. Participant's body composition was assessed via Dual-energy X-ray Absorptiometry (Hologic QDR Series Discovery A, Bedfored, MA). Height and mass measurements were taken according to the anthropometric profile recommended by the International Society for the advancement of Kinantropometry (ISAK)[19] using a Stadiometer (Seca, Germany) and electronic weighing scales (Seca, Hamburg, Germany). Blood pressure and resting heart rate were measured using an automatic upper arm blood pressure monitor (Dynamap, Critikon, UK) following a 5 min period of seated rest. Two measurements were recorded and an average calculated from this data for the final recorded measurement. Blood samples were obtained from the antecubital vein in 2 mL syringes without heparin. Plasma from centrifuged samples was collected and stored at −20 °C until subsequent analysis. High-density lipoprotein (HDL), low-density lipoprotein (LDL), triglycerides and total cholesterol were determined flourometrically on an automatic analyser (RX Daytona, Randox Laboratory, Antrim, UK). All samples were measured in duplicate following completion of the 12-week programme using the same commercially available enzymatic spectrophotometric assays (RX Daytona Analyser, Randox Laboratories, Antrim, UK). Co-efficient of variation for these assay kits were 1.47, 1.80, 3.29 and 3.73% for HDL, LDL, triglycerides and total cholesterol, respectively.

Statistics

Data are presented as means ± standard deviation (SD). All data were assessed for the assumption of normality using the Shapiro–Wilks test for normality of distribution. Mauchly's test of sphericity was performed on all data to assess for the assumption of sphericity. However, no corrections were required following these assessments. Within-group data for all variables for pre-, mid- and post-testing (Weeks – 1, 6 and 12) were evaluated by one-way analysis of variance on repeated measures (ANOVA). The level of statistical significance was set at $p < 0.05$. When a significant effect was detected, data were subsequently analysed using Bonferonni corrected pair-wise comparison post hoc test. All statistical analyses were carried out using SPSS Statistical Analysis Software (SPSS® Version 15.0.01 for Windows®, Chicago, Illinois, USA).

Results

Physiological response to training

Average HR during sessions across the 12 weeks was 138 ± 7 beats min^{-1}. This corresponded to around $75 \pm 4\%$ HR_{max}. Average time spent $>90\%$ HR_{max} for each session was 13 ± 7 min (Table 1), corresponding to 15% of training time. Mean RPE for the sessions was 6 ± 1 (VAS 1–10). These data gave an RPE_{load} of 475 ± 71 (Table 1). Average HR during the warm-up, technical practice, skills/possession practice and SSG were 67 ± 6, 71 ± 4, 76 ± 5 and $82 \pm 7\%$ HR_{max}, respectively (Figure 1). Figure 2 provides an individual insight into the sessional HR response for a typical training session.

Blood pressure and resting heart rate

No differences ($p = 1.00$) were observed for RHR between weeks-1 and -6. Resting heart rate did, however, change ($p = 0.008$) from 87 ± 22 beats min^{-1} at week-6, to 72 ± 17 beats min^{-1} at week-12 (Table 2 and Figure 3). No changes were observed in resting systolic ($p = 0.711$) or diastolic ($p = 0.824$) blood pressure following 12 weeks of training (Table 2).

Body composition and blood analysis

No changes occurred over 12-weeks of training for total mass ($p = 0.144$), fat ($p = 0.173$) and lean mass ($p = 0.484$), bone mineral density (BMD) ($p = 0.199$) and %body fat ($p = 0.098$) (Table 2). Similarly, no changes were observed over 12-

Table 1.   Mean ± SD data ($n = 9$) for session duration, RPE, RPE Load, and HR training data for 12 weeks of football training. Mean HR data are the mean of both sessions during the week.

Week	Mean session duration (min)	RPE (VAS1–10)	RPE load	Overall mean heart rate (beats min^{-1})	% HR_{max}	Time >90% HR_{max} (min)
Week 1	73 ± 30	7 ± 0	511	136 ± 24	75 ± 3	10 ± 6
Week 2	74 ± 35	6 ± 1	444	135 ± 16	74 ± 3	2 ± 2
Week 3	104 ± 7	5 ± 1	521	145 ± 20	79 ± 3	21 ± 18
Week 4	93 ± 0	6 ± 0	558	132 ± 18	72 ± 3	10 ± 15
Week 5	89 ± 1	6 ± 2	534	136 ± 23	74 ± 3	15 ± 15
Week 6	80 ± 37	5 ± 1	400	133 ± 24	73 ± 3	8 ± 11
Week 7	92 ± 4	6 ± 2	552	148 ± 22	81 ± 3	21 ± 18
Week 8	99 ± 2	4 ± 0	396	141 ± 21	77 ± 3	17 ± 15
Week 9	92 ± 11	5 ± 1	460	132 ± 19	72 ± 3	14 ± 12
Week 10	100 ± 0	4 ± 0	400	140 ± 25	76 ± 3	14 ± 15
Week 11	92 ± 3	6 ± 1	552	143 ± 19	78 ± 3	12 ± 15
Week 12	53 ± 0	7 ± 0	371	132 ± 24	72 ± 3	7 ± 7
Overall mean ± SD	88 ± 18	6 ± 1	475 ±71	138 ± 7	75 ± 3	13 ± 7

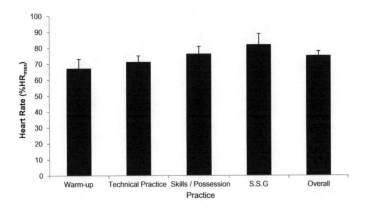

Figure 1.   Mean ± SD HR values (%HR$_{max}$) for activity breakdown during football sessions.

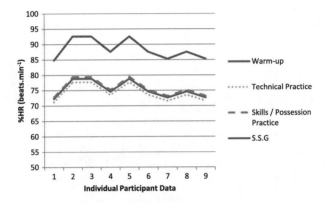

Figure 2.   Individual HR data for a single session within the programme, highlighting the variability between participants and HR increase during the SSG.

weeks of training for blood lipid markers, including HDL ($p = 0.187$), LDL ($p = 0.487$), triglycerides ($p = 0.541$) and total cholesterol ($p = 0.108$) (Table 3).

Discussion

The primary aim of the current investigation was to examine markers of health before and after a 12-week FitC health programme. The main finding was that 12 weeks of a recreational community based football training programme elicited little or no changes in physiological markers of health as reflected by HR, blood pressure, body composition and blood lipid profile. However, it could be suggested that the programme was successful in maintaining health, as the participants' baseline data suggests that they were not especially unhealthy. The failure to find positive changes in health may be consequence of the myriad of problems associated with the delivery of such programmes within the community based setting (e.g. participant attendance). They may also be a result of the relatively low exercise intensity associated with the sessions included in the intervention. This intensity is probably a direct result of the organization of the activities within the session. This may highlight the need for better coach education training for the delivery of community programmes.

31

Table 2. Mean ± SD group body composition, blood pressure and resting heart rate for Weeks 1, 6 and 12.

	Week 1	Week 6	Week 12
Body composition			
Mass (kg)	75.4 ± 13.7	74.7 ± 13.7	74.0 ± 14.7
BMI	24.85	24.62	24.39
BMD (g cm^2)	1.240 ± 0.135	1.247 ± 0.124	1.194 ± 0.093
Fat mass (kg)*	13.9 ± 6.4	14.7 ± 7.3	13.8 ± 6.3
Lean mass (kg)*	54.0 ± 8.9	53.6 ± 8.3	55.0 ± 9.7
Total fat (%)*	19.2 ± 5.8	20.2 ± 6.4	18.9 ± 5.6
Blood pressure			
Systolic BP (mmHg)	134 ± 14	134 ± 12	131 ± 11
Diastolic BP (mmHg)	76 ± 13	78 ± 9	79 ± 9
RHR (beats min^{-1})	88 ± 20	87 ± 22	72 ± 17[#]**

Note: BMD – bone mineral density, BMI – body mass index, BP – blood pressure, RHR – resting heart rate.
*Indicates subtotal value (i.e. excluding head).
**Indicates significant difference from Week 6.
[#]Significant difference from Week 1.

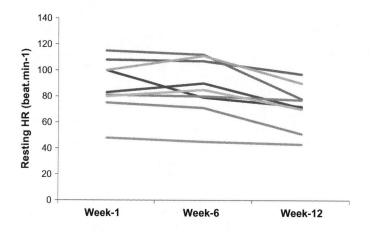

Figure 3. Individual RHR pre, during and post the 12-week training programme.

Table 3. Mean ± SD blood lipid values for Weeks 1, 6 and 12.

	Week 1	Week 6	Week 12
Cholesterol (mmol L^{-1})	5.28 ± 0.83	5.28 ± 0.49	5.31 ± 0.79
Triglycerides (mmol L^{-1})	1.85 ± 0.42	2.04 ± 0.43	1.83 ± 0.40
HDL (mmol L^{-1})	1.10 ± 0.15	1.13 ± 0.22	1.12 ± 0.20
LDL (mmol L^{-1})	3.53 ± 0.95	3.50 ± 0.81	3.46 ± 0.92
HDL/LDL ratio	0.85 ± 0.41	0.95 ± 0.57	0.79 ± 0.36

The training programme included in the intervention had limited impact on a selected range of markers of health in our HTR population. No changes were observed in blood pressure, body composition (including; fat mass, lean mass, %

body fat and BMD) and blood lipid profile. The findings in the current investigation are in contrast to previous research that indicated that recreational football training, with an approximate intensity of 80–85% generated during a 60–120 min session 2–3 times per week, was effective in reducing blood pressure. For example, previous investigations[20] have observed reductions in systolic and diastolic blood pressure of 8 and 5 mm Hg, respectively, following 12-weeks of training. Recent studies have also typically observed reductions in total mass, fat mass and % body fat as well as increases in leg muscle mass and BMD following a period of recreational football training.[21] These data are also in contrast to our findings. Resting HR was the only variable to decrease following 12 weeks of recreational football training (Table 2) in the current investigation. The decrease in resting HR as observed in previous studies[22] may reflect a reduction in sympathetic outflow and thereby reduced systemic vascular restrictions. Regardless of the lack of physiological change observed, it cannot be ascertained if the programme resulted in other adaptations in either behavioural and/or psychological characteristics. Such changes have previously been seen in other investigations,[23] though were not measured here.

Mean weekly time spent above 90% HR_{max} equated to 13 ± 7 min throughout the 12 training weeks. This may have been thought to be sufficient to induce a positive health increase as previous studies[24] demonstrate, although still lower than findings within a street soccer programme[25] that resulted in 21 ± 12 min above 90% HR_{max}. The lack of significance amongst the physiological variables could partially be attributed to the depletion of the statistical power due to the withdrawal of 11 participants from the original group of 20. This may have decreased the likelihood of any statistical difference from several of the variables measured, as positive improvements are clear but not to significance. This, and the lack of a control group, is a clear limitation of this investigation. Another possible explanation for the lack of health benefits observed following the programme may be linked to the overall exercise intensity achieved during the sessions. The overall average intensity of the football sessions conducted throughout the 12-week programme was $75 \pm 4\%$ HR_{max}. This is considerably lower than reported in recent research that has utilized a more controlled exercise prescription such as SSG.[26] The main disparity in the overall exercise intensity within our investigation seemed to have occurred as a consequence of the structure of the session, more specifically the inclusion of football drills and technical practices. Average HRs during technical practice and skills/possession practice were 71 ± 4 and $76 \pm 5\%$ HR_{max}, respectively (Figure 1). This is lower than the 82% HR_{max} associated with the SSGs completed at the end of the session. The intensity of exercise is thought to act as a key primer for any physiological adaptations associated with chronic training programmes.[27] The previous research discussed[28] would suggest that an overall intensity between 80 and 85% HR_{max} would induce adaptation within a healthy population, similar to those described in the current investigation. Therefore, it appears that the inclusion of technically orientated football drills may have lowered the overall exercise intensity of the session and limited the time that each participant was required to work at near maximal levels of cardiovascular stress. This may suggest that programmes that do not create high physiological loads may not be effective in eliciting positive health gains. Thus, the absence of change in physiological markers of health observed in the current study could be explained by an insufficient training stimulus. An additional factor that may have explained the lack of effectiveness of the programme was the reduced average duration of the sessions (88 ± 18 min, see Table 1) when compared to scheduled completion time of 120 min. This discrepancy was accredited to poor timekeeping of the HTR population, which severely restricted the ability of the coach to run the session for the appropriate duration.

Exercise conducted as part of community-based football health programmes may therefore, need to be more highly controlled from a physiological viewpoint in order to elicit the desired adaptations that may lead to improvements in health status. Beneficial adaptations to the exercise incorporated in such programmes could include a greater reliance on SSG's or a manipulation of any technically orientated football drill included within the session to increase the physiological load. For example, the size of area, number of players and the exercise to rest ratio are all important determinants of the overall physiological stress associated with the training stimulus[29] that could be manipulated by the coach to improve the fitness outcomes of the session. Furthermore, SSGs have resulted in lower RPE values than jogging, interval training and strength training.[30] Providing more evidence for the use of SSGs. The current investigation found a higher RPE responses compared to previous research[30], although this may be due to the inclusions of training drills, and may have affected participant retention. There is also a need for further research to investigate the optimal dose response for beneficial health adaptations. It could be speculated that training twice per week for 60–120 min would be suffice, although this may be dependent on the baseline health of the population undertaking the programme. There is a lack of understanding as to the effect of shorter football training or SSG sessions conducted and maintaining higher exercise intensities. This may be appropriate for populations that are not unhealthy, such as a more aggressive and intense programme can be prescribed, although more research is needed to investigate this hypothesis. Another potential aspect to consider is the development of appropriate standards of coach education for practitioners involved in this type of programme. Typically, the coaches that lead community based programmes complete the same educational programmes as coaches who focus on the development of players from a technical and tactical perspective. This type of syllabus may not be suitable for the delivery of a knowledge base that equips individuals to deliver football sessions that are aimed at providing a suitable physiological intensity to improve markers of health. This study illustrates that the intensity of the session is paramount in providing beneficial health gains for participants, which may require the use of appropriate measures for the monitoring of the intensity to ensure that the coaches are providing a sufficient load to generate the physiologic and metabolic adaptations. However, the coaches may also need to be mindful of the psychological issues that may impact the participation and potential behavioural change. It is important that the training does not simply become fitness-based drills to increase intensity, but retain the inclusion of football-based drills and SSGs carefully designed to generate sufficient intensity, as these have shown to provide increases in motivation that can increase physical activity compliance.

In conclusion, community-based football projects endorsed by elite teams may be successful at engaging those from HTR populations and important to combat increasing levels of physical inactivity in the general population and associated levels of obesity and cardiovascular diseases. However, the current study suggests that exercise administered during these programmes may not be efficient in promoting positive health changes, although it was successful in maintaining health over the 12-week intervention. As the HTR population were not necessarily unhealthy, more time could be prescribed for SSGs that may not only increase intensity, but also lower RPE, yet maintain participation. It is important for long-term success that the education of participants and healthy lifestyle messages endorsed by such programmes are supported by measurable positive health adaptations. As such, careful consideration needs to be taken when planning training programmes. The completion of a suitable amount of exercise at a high intensity would seem to be an important component of such a planning process. This may necessitate the improved training and education programmes of personal that are required to deliver the programmes.

Acknowledgements

The authors would like to express their gratitude to the participants of the Premier League Health programme and the staff of Everton in the Community and Everton Football Club.

Disclosure statement

No potential conflict of interest was reported by the authors.

Notes

1. Pringle et al., 'Effect of a National Programme of Men's Health Delivered in English Premier League Football Clubs'.
2. World Health Organisation, 'Social Determinants of Health'.
3. Faugier and Sargeant, 'Sampling Hard to Reach Populations'.
4. Witty and White, *The Tackling Men's Health Evaluation Study*.
5. Randers et al., 'Positive Performance and Health Effects of a Football Training Program over 12-weeks can be Maintained over a 1-year period with Reduced Training Frequency'; Krustrup et al., 'Recreational Soccer is an Effective Health Promoting Activity for Untrained Men'.
6. Wilkins and Baker, *Getting it Sorted: A Policy Programme for Men's Health*.
7. Gough, 'The Psychology of Men's Health: Maximising Masculine Capital'.
8. Krustrup et al., 'Effects on Training Status and Health Profile of Prolonged Participation in Recreational Football: Heart Rate (HR) Response to Recreational Training and Match-play'; Krustrup et al., 'Recreational Soccer is an Effective Health Promoting Activity for Untrained Men'; Bangsbo et al., 'Performance Enhancements and Muscular Adaptations of a 16-week Recreational Football Intervention for Untrained Women'; Anderson et al., 'Football as a Treatment for Hypertension in Untrained 30–55 year-old men: A Prospective Randomized Study'; and Randers et al., 'Positive Performance and Health Effects of a Football Training Program over 12-weeks can be Maintained over a 1-year Period with Reduced Training Frequency'.
9. Krustrup et al., 'Recreational Soccer is an Effective Health Promoting Activity for Untrained Men'.
10. Anderson et al., 'Football as a Treatment for Hypertension in Untrained 30–55 year-old Men: A Prospective Randomized Study'.
11. Randers et al., 'Positive Performance and Health Effects of a Football Training Program over 12-weeks can be Maintained over a 1-year Period with Reduced Training Frequency'.
12. Krustrup et al., 'Muscle Adaptations and Performance Enhancements of Soccer Training for Untrained Men'.
13. Krustrup et al., 'Effects on Training Status and Health Profile of Prolonged Participation in Recreational Football: Heart Rate Response to Recreational Training and Match-play'; Krustrup et al., 'Recreational Soccer is an Effective Health Promoting Activity for Untrained Men'; Bangsbo et al., 'Performance Enhancements and Muscular

Adaptations of a 16-week Recreational Football Intervention for Untrained Women'; Anderson et al., 'Football as a Treatment for Hypertension in Untrained 30–55 year-old Men: A Prospective Randomized Study'; and Randers et al., 'Positive Performance and Health Effects of a Football Training Program over 12-weeks can be Maintained over a 1-year Period with Reduced Training Frequency'.

14. Golay et al., 'Taking Small Steps towards Targets – Perspectives for Clinical Practice in Diabetes, Cardiometabolic Disorders and Beyond', (2013).
15. Yates and Williams, 'The Microstructure of Practice in Soccer: A Comparison of Duration and Frequency of Practice'.
16. Foster et al., 'Effects of Specific versus Cross-training on Running Performance'.
17. Ibid.
18. Imellizzeri et al., 'Use of RPE-based Training Load in Soccer'.
19. Marfell-Jones et al., 'International Standards for Anthropometrical Assessment'.
20. Krustrup et al., 'Recreational Soccer is an Effective Health Promoting Activity for Untrained Men'.
21. Bangsbo et al., 'Performance Enhancements and Muscular Adaptations of a 16-week Recreational Football Intervention for Untrained Women'; Krustrup et al., 'Recreational Soccer is an Effective Health Promoting Activity for Untrained Men'; 'Krustrup et al., 'Muscle Adaptations and Performance Enhancements of Soccer Training for Untrained Men'; and Randers et al., 'Positive Performance and Health Effects of a Football Training Program over 12-weeks can be Maintained over a 1-year Period with Reduced Training Frequency'.
22. Krustrup et al., 'Recreational Soccer is an Effective Health Promoting Activity for Untrained Men'; Anderson et al., 'Football as a Treatment for Hypertension in Untrained 30–55 year-old Men: A Prospective Randomized Study'; and Randers et al., 'Positive Performance and Health Effects of a Football Training Program over 12-weeks can be Maintained over a 1-year Period with Reduced Training Frequency'.
23. Pringle et al., Effect of a National Programme of Men's Health Delivered in English Premier League Football Clubs'.
24. Nybo et al., 'High-intensity Training versus Traditional Exercise Interventions for Promoting Health'; Krustrup et al., 'Recreational Soccer is an Effective Health Promoting Activity for Untrained Men'.
25. Randers et al., 'Short-term Street Soccer Improves Fitness and Cardiovascular Health Status of Homeless Men'.
26. Bangsbo et al., 'Performance Enhancements and Muscular Adaptations of a 16-week Recreational Football Intervention for Untrained Women'; Krustrup et al., 'Recreational Soccer is an Effective Health Promoting Activity for Untrained Men'; Krustrup et al., 'Muscle Adaptations and Performance Enhancements of Soccer Training for Untrained Men'; and Randers et al., 'Positive Performance and Health Effects of a Football Training Program over 12-weeks can be Maintained over a one-year Period with Reduced Training Frequency'.
27. Nybo et al., 'High-intensity Training versus Traditional Exercise Interventions for Promoting Health'.
28. Bangsbo et al., 'Performance Enhancements and Muscular Adaptations of a 16-week Recreational Football Intervention for Untrained Women'; Krustrup et al., 'Recreational Soccer is an Effective Health Promoting Activity for Untrained Men'; Krustrup et al., 'Muscle Adaptations and Performance Enhancements of Soccer Training for Untrained Men'; and Randers et al., 'Positive Performance and Health Effects of a Football Training Program over 12-weeks can be Maintained over a 1-year Period with Reduced Training Frequency'.
29. Köklüet et al., 'Comparison of the Physiological Responses to Different Small-sided Games in Elite Young Soccer Players'.
30. Elbe et al., 'Experiencing Flow in Different Types of Physical Activity Intervention Programs: Three Randomized Studies'.

References

Andersen, L.J., M.B. Randers, K. Westh, D. Martone, P.R. Hansen, A. Junge, J. Dvorak, J. Bangsbo, and P. Krustrup. 'Football as a Treatment for Hypertension in Untrained 30–55 Year-old Men: A Prospective Randomized Study'. *Scandinavian Journal of Medicine & Science in Sports* 20 (2010): 98–102.

Bangsbo, J., J.J. Nielsen, M. Mohr, M.B. Randers, B.R. Krustrup, J. Brito, L. Nybo, and P. Krustrup. 'Performance Enhancements and Muscular Adaptations of a 16-week Recreational Football Intervention for Untrained Women'. *Scandinavian Journal of Medicine & Science in Sports* 20 (2010): 24–30.

Bergeron, M.F. 'Improving Health through Youth Sports: Is Participation Enough?' *New Directions for Youth Development* 115 (2007): 27–41.

Elbe, A.M., K. Strahler, P. Krustrup, J. Wikman, and R. Stelter. 'Experiencing Flow in Different Types of Physical Activity Intervention Programs: Three Randomized Studies'. *Scandinavian Journal of Medicine & Science in Sports* 20, supplement (2010): 111–7.

Faugier, J., and M. Sargeant. 'Sampling Hard to Reach Populations'. *Journal of Advanced Nursing* 26 (1997): 790–7.

Foster, C., L. Hector, R. Welsh, M. Schrager, M.A. Green, and A.C. Snyder. 'Effects of Specific versus Cross-training on Running Performance'. *European Journal of Applied Physiology and Occupational Physiology* 70 (1995): 367–72.

Golay, A., E. Brock, R. Gabriel, T. Konrad, N. Lalic, M. Laville, G. Mingrone et al. 'Taking Small Steps towards Targets – Perspectives for Clinical Practice in Diabetes, Cardiometabolic Disorders and beyond'. *International Journal of Clinical Practice* 67 (2013): 322–32.

Gough, B. 'The Psychology of Men's Health: Maximizing Masculine Capital'. *Health Psychology* 32, no. 1 (2013): 1–4.

Helgerud, J., L.C. Engen, Ulrik Wisloff, and J. Hoff. 'Aerobic Endurance Training Improves Soccer Performance'. *Medicine and Science in Sports and Exercise* 33 (2001): 1925–31.

Impellizzeri, F.M., E. Rampinini, A.J. Coutts, A. Sassi, and S.M. Marcora. 'Use of RPE-based Training Load in Soccer'. *Medicine and Science in Sports and Exercise* 36 (2004): 1042–7.

Köklü, Y., A. Aşçi, F.U. Koçak, U. Alemdaroğlu, and U. Dündar. 'Comparison of the Physiological Responses to Different Small-sided Games in Elite Young Soccer Players'. *Journal of Strength and Conditioning Research* 25 (2011): 1522–8.

Krustrup, P., and J. Bangsbo. 'Physiological Demands of Top-class Soccer Refereeing in Relation to Physical Capacity: Effect of Intense Intermittent Exercise Training'. *Journal of Sports Science* 19 (2001): 811–91.

Krustrup, P., J.F. Christensen, M.B. Randers, H. Pedersen, E. Sundstrup, M.D. Jakobsen, B.R. Krustrup et al. 'Muscle Adaptations and Performance Enhancements of Soccer Training for Untrained Men'. *European Journal of Applied Physiology* 108 (2010): 1247–58.

Krustrup, P., P.R. Hansen, M.B. Randers, L. Nybo, D. Martone, L.J. Andersen, L.T. Bune, A. Junge, and J. Bangsbo. 'Beneficial Effects of Recreational Football on the Cardiovascular Risk Profile in Untrained Premenopausal Women'. *Scandinavian Journal of Medicine & Science in Sports* 20 (2010): 40–9.

Krustrup, P., J.J. Nielsen, B. Krustrup, J.F. Christensen, H. Pedersen, M.B. Randers, P. Aagaard, A.M. Petersen, L. Nybo, and J. Bangsbo. 'Recreational Soccer is an Effective Health Promoting Activity for Untrained Men'. *British Journal of Sports Medicine* 43 (2009): 825–31.

Krustrup, B.R., I. Rollo, J.N. Nielsen, and P. Krustrup. 'Effects on Training Status and Health Profile of Prolonged Participation in Recreational Football: Heart Rate Response to Recreational Training and Match-play'. *Journal of Sports Science and Medicine* 6 (2007): 116–7.

Lee, I.M., and P.J. Skerrett. 'Physical Activity and All-cause Mortality: What is the Dose–response Relation?' *Medicine and Science in Sports and Exercise* 34 (2001): 592–5.

Marfell-Jones, M., T. Olds, A. Stewart, and J.E.L. Carter. 'International Standards for Anthropometrical Assessment'. *Potchesfstroom: International Society for the Advancement of Kinanthtopometry* 2 (2006): 1–137.

Nybo, L., E. Sundstrup, M.D. Jakobsen, M. Mohr, T. Hornstrup, L. Simonsen, J. Bülow et al. 'High-intensity Training versus Traditional Exercise Interventions for Promoting Health'. *Medicine and Science in Sports and Exercise* 42 (2010): 1951–8.

Pringle, A., S. Zwolinsky, J. McKenna, A. Daly-Smith, S. Robertson, and A. White. 'Effect of a National Programme of Men's Health Delivered in English Premier League Football Clubs'. *Public Health* 127 (2013): 18–26.

Pringle, A., S. Zwolinsky, A. Smith, S. Robertson, J. McKenna, and A. White. 'The Pre-adoption Demographic and Health Profiles of Men Participating in a Programme of Men's Health Delivered in English Premier League Football Clubs'. *Public Health* 125 (2011): 411–6.

Randers, M.B., J.J. Nielsen, B.R. Krustrup, E. Sundstrup, M.D. Jakobsen, L. Nybo, J. Dvorak, J. Bangsbo, and P. Krustrup. 'Positive Performance and Health Effects of a Football Training Program over 12-weeks Can Be Maintained over a 1-year Period with Reduced Training Frequency'. *Scandinavian Journal of Medicine & Science in Sports* 20 (2010): 80–9.

Randers, M.P., J. Petersen, L.J. Andersen, B.R. Krustrup, T. Hornstrup, J.J. Nielsen, M. Nordentoft, and P. Krustrup. 'Short-term Street Soccer Improves Fitness and Cardiovascular Health Status of Homeless Men'. *European Journal of Applied Physiology* 112 (2012): 2097–106.

Wilkins, D., and P. Baker. *Getting It Sorted: A Policy Programme for Men's Health.* London: Men's Health Forum, 2003.

Witty, K., and A. White. *The Tackling Men's Health Evaluation Study.* Leeds: Centre for Men's Health, Leeds Metropolitan University, 2010.

World Health Organisation. 'Social Determinants of Health'. 2003. http://www.who.int/social_determinants/publications/en/ (accessed July 2013).

Yates, I.S., and A.M. Williams. 'The Microstructure of Practice in Soccer: A Comparison of Duration and Frequency of Practice'. In *Science and Football VI, Proceedings of the 6th World Congress in Science and Football*, ed. T. Reilly and F. Korkusuz, 437–41. Turkey: Antalya, 2008.

Evaluating conflict mitigation and health improvement through soccer: a two-year study of Mifalot's 'United Soccer for Peace' programme

Tal Litvak-Hirsch[a], Yair Galily[b] and Michael Leitner[c]

[a]Management and Conflict Resolution Program, Ben Gurion University of the Negev, Beersheva, Israel; [b]Sammy Ofer School of Communications, Interdisciplinary Center (IDC) Herzliya, Herzliya, Israel; [c]Department of Recreation, Hospitality, and Parks Management, California State University, Chico, CA, USA

War not only has a direct impact on health through its direct physical consequences but also through the stress experienced by all those directly and indirectly affected by it. Therefore, conflict mitigation efforts can make a significant positive impact on health. In Israel, a country that has experienced a great deal of conflict, utilizing sports to foster peaceful relations and coexistence is an idea that has gained popularity in recent years. The aim of this article is to examine in-depth, using social psychological theoretical lenses one project, Mifalot's 'United Soccer for Peace' soccer coaching certification course. The course trains adult Arab and Jewish soccer coaches in mixed groups, as well as to teach them peace education values and tools. This study examined the successes and challenges of this project in contributing to conflict mitigation and health improvement. Some of the specific questions addressed were: Why did many Arab participants leave the project in its early stages? What can be done to improve this project and similar projects like this in the future? There were 63 coaches, Israeli Arabs and Jews interviewed. In general, the results provide evidence that sports can contribute to coexistence and improved health with the right theoretical understanding, planning and organization. Achievements as well as challenges of the project are discussed and recommendations for improvement and implementation to other conflict areas are suggested.

Introduction

There have been a number of attempts in Israel in recent years to utilize the power of soccer [or football] to bring Arabs and Jews together in order to improve relations and make peace in the region a possibility. This study examines the effectiveness of one particular programme, Mifalot's 'United Soccer for Peace' in reaching this goal. A growing number of studies from around the world[1] demonstrate the potential for the use of sport as a vehicle to promote mutual understanding, reconciliation and coexistence in deeply divided societies. In Israel, there is growing interest in the role of sports programmes in conflict mitigation.[2] However, there is relatively little research, which examines the effects of these sports programmes in Israel. Most of the research conducted in Israel in this field is quantitative and addresses issues of attitude changes, development of local commitment and leadership, and improving sports programming.[3] The aim of this paper is to examine in-depth, using qualitative

39

methods, one project, Mifalot's 'United Soccer for Peace'. This three-year programme attempts to train and certify 25 Arab and 25 Jewish soccer coaches each year in mixed groups, as well as to teach them peace education values and tools. The certified coaches then apply for small grants to conduct programmes in their communities that bring together Arab and Jewish children for soccer activities.

The following section provides a review of existing views and transnational research on the issue of sports as a facilitator of peaceful relations and coexistence is presented, followed by a description of the current relationship between Jews and Arabs citizens of Israel. This is culminated by suggesting the contact hypothesis[4] as a theorizing anchor for sports programmes, which are aimed to enhance coexistence and through the provision of recent studies that have been conducted in Israel in the last few years in the area of sports and coexistence.

Sports as a facilitator of peaceful relations and coexistence in the world

Following the advice of Kidd,[5] which outlined for practitioners and policymakers to gain knowledge of the circumstances under which sport results in positive outcomes for gender relations, disability inclusion, youth development, mental health, peace and conflict resolution for various populations, numerous organizations, with the support of several international sports federations, NGOs and enthusiastic endorsement by the United Nations and its agencies and partners. A new, worldwide 'sport for development and peace movement' in 2008 emerged.[6] In 2010, the *American Institute of Peace* organized a 'Sports and Peace-building Symposium', which, according to the organisers, was the first academic event focusing exclusively on the intersection of sport and peace-building organized by an institution not directly involved in the field. According to Tuohey and Cognate, though a modest event in the peace-building world as a whole, the Symposium marked a significant milestone for sport-for-peace practitioners – the first step to establishing a theoretically rigorous and empirically sound framework for sport-based peace-building that can help develop policy support, synchronize practitioner efforts and ultimately aid the efforts of all those working to prevent, mitigate or end conflict worldwide.[7]

Levermore,[8] tried to sharpen the desired outcomes of sport-for-development and peace organizations. Among these outcomes, one can count conflict resolution and intercultural understanding; building physical, social and community infrastructure; raising awareness, particularly through education; empowerment; direct impact on physical and psychological health and general welfare; economic development and poverty alleviation. Such Functionalist perspective long rooted in the work of Merton, Parsons and their successors,[9] all share a view that suggests that sport is used to promote common values held essential for the integration and development of a society. Thus, 'sports for peace' programmes help to maintain social order. They focus on participation and positive outcomes for individuals and society, and increase opportunities to foster individual development. Such belief clearly underpins the view of sport as an apolitical, neutral and inherently integrative set of social practices that can deliver a wide range of positive outcomes.

Probably the broadest view about the potential of sports in the area of conflict mitigation stems from Sugden's work.[10] Drawing from the role played by sport in South Africa before and after apartheid and his own experiences, garnered over more than two decades of conducting research and leading sport-based intervention initiatives in Northern Ireland and Israel, he argues that sport is intrinsically value neutral and under carefully managed circumstances it can make a positive if modest contribution to peace building. In a study in Sri Lanka, Schulenkorf[11] found that if strategically designed, sports programmes can promote the establishment of friendships and inclusive social identities among diverse populations. Another study, conducted in Russia with victims of terrorism[12] found that the quality of the staff and design of the programmes were key factors related to the effectiveness of football-based interventions in promoting peace.

Jews and Arabs in Israel

Israel is home to a widely diverse population from many different ethnic, religious, cultural and social backgrounds; a new society with ancient roots, which is still coalescing and developing today.[13] There is great concern over relations between Israeli Arabs and Jews. The Arabs are about 20% of Israel population and most of them are Muslims.[14] Results from a recent survey[15] suggested that 48% of the Arab citizens claimed that they are not content with their quality of life in Israel and 29% claim that they do not want to have Jewish friends. As for the Jews, 58% claimed that they are afraid of gaining control of Arabs due to their high birth rate and 79% agreed that Arabs should have the rights to live as a minority with full rights. However, 58% do not want to have an Arab manager. These results are somewhat better than past surveys, which suggested that approximately 43% of Israeli Jews have a negative view of Israeli Arabs and only 7% have a positive views.[16] Moreover, Israeli Jews expressed stereotypes such as Arabs being primitive (38%), violent (38%), and dirty (32%). Perhaps, most striking are the statistics cited by Smooha indicating that approximately 66% of Israeli Arabs agree that it is impossible to trust most Jews, and approximately 66% of Israeli Jews agree that it is impossible to trust most Arabs in Israel.[17] Thus, programmes that bring together Israeli Arabs and Jews in a positive atmosphere can potentially play an important role in improving relations between Israel's Arabs and Jews. Deteriorating relations between Israel's Arabs and Jews would be harmful to the health and well-being of the nation and its efforts to make peace with its Arab neighbours.

Sports programmes that enhance coexistence in Israel – theory and practice

Many peace coexistence programmes that involve initiated meeting and collaboration between Jews and Arabs are based on two main social psychological theoretical anchors. One is the work of Tajfel's on social identities.[18] Tagfel and Turner claim that representations of 'the other' and 'the self', and the changes that occur over time concerning these representations, play a central role in the creation of personal and collective identity. Over the life course, one meets different significant others who influence us, as we influence them. In turn people construct their identity in relation to those others. The second hypothesis that plays a central role in initiating programmes that consists of mixed groups of Jews and Arabs is Alport's 'Contact Hypothesis'.[19] The premise of Alport's theory states that under appropriate conditions interpersonal contact is one of the most effective ways to reduce prejudice between majority and minority group members. If one has the opportunity to communicate with others, they are able to understand and appreciate different points of views involving their way of life. As a result of new appreciation and understanding, prejudice should diminish. Issues of stereotyping, prejudice and discrimination are commonly occurring issues between rival groups. Alport's proposal was that properly managed contact between the groups should reduce these problems and lead to better interactions between members of the groups. However, research suggests[20] that in order to obtain beneficial effects, the situation must include these criteria:

(1) *Equal Status of both groups:* Members of the groups should have similar backgrounds, qualities and characteristics. For example, it is better to have participants of similar socio-economic background and ages, to not have differences in these areas which could serve as an additional challenge to encouraging positive interaction between members of the groups.

(2) *Common Goals:* both groups work on a problem/task and share this as a common goal.

(3) *Intergroup Cooperation:* both groups must work together for their common goals without competition.

(4) *Support of authorities, law or customs:* some authority that both groups acknowledge and define social norms that support the contact and interactions between the groups and members and

(5) *Personal Interaction:* the contact situation needs to involve informal, personal interaction with outgroup members. Members of the conflicting groups need to mingle with one another. Without these criteria they learn very little about each other and cross-group friendships do not occur.[21]

Following these theoretical understandings, some sports programmes that are aimed to enhance coexistence and contribute to peace building have evolved in Israel in recent years. An example of a sports programme contributing to peace building in Israel is 'Football for Peace'. Football for Peace is a grassroots, sports-based coexistence programme that tries to improve relations between Arabs and Jews in Israel through soccer, across 33 communities in Israel, mostly in the Galilee region.[22] Research on this programme identified several key positive dimensions that promote better intercommunity relations, such as developing local commitment and leadership and improving sports programming.[23] Three more recent research studies on the effects of integrated sports programmes with Arabs and Jews in Israel were conducted in 2011–2012. Two of the studies were based on programmes organized by 'The Peres Center for Peace' and by 'Mifalot'. These were delivered to children ages 8–15, providing them with monthly joint sports activities throughout the academic year. The attitudes of the children in these studies towards 'the other' changed positively during the year.[24] One other study concerning The Friendship Games was delivered with young adults and was an intensive one week event in which all participants stay at the same hotel, participate in a variety of activities together, and have many opportunities for informal joint activity (e.g. going out on the town together late at night). The research results indicate participation in events such as The Friendship Games have positive implications for both Arabs and Jews.[25]

The aim of the current research is to explore one programme, Mifalot's 'United Soccer for Peace' soccer coach's certification course, which is aimed to train adult Arab and Jewish soccer coaches in mixed groups, as well as to teach them peace education values and tools. The following questions were asked: What are the successes and challenges of such programmes that are aimed to integrate sports and peace education within mixed groups of Jews and Arabs in Israel? Why did many

Arab participants leave the programme in its early stages? What can be done to improve this project and similar programme like this in the future? How can more Arabs be recruited for these programmes?

Background on the Mifalot 'United Soccer for Peace' project

'United Soccer for Peace' is a three-year programme aimed at creating an environment conducive to implanting a movement for social change through soccer. To achieve this goal, in the first phase of the project, the Mifalot and their partners recruit a total of 150 participants (50 per year), both Jews and Arabs, and provide training. The training provides participants with certification as soccer coaches, peace activists and community leaders. The process of recruitment was held through the media and sport clubs. The opportunity to receive certification as a soccer coach at a low cost or no cost is a major incentive for most of the participants to choose to join the programme. The training course takes eight months, with meetings on a weekly basis as well as a two-day 'peace seminar' in Givaat Haviva. In the second phase, the participants are able to apply these skills as coaches to approximately 11,000 youth (6000 youth + 5000 micro-grant initiative participants) who will learn these values of conflict mitigation, coexistence and community activism. Mifalot attempts to promote sustainability, self-sufficiency and expanding social influence by offering micro-grants to participants to continue in their roles as coaches. Creating social change in the face of such intense and deep conflict requires creating the proper environment for change, growth and sustainability. Mifalot believes that if they can create a group of educated peace activists and skilled leaders that enter society, first, as coaches and youth leaders, and, later, as productive members of society dedicated to community activism, then their efforts will spread values of peace and community involvement to jumpstart lasting social change. This approach aims to empower both the individual and the local community through two methodologies, peace education and internal community development. Combining soccer with this approach aspires to unite populations in conflict and creates self-sustaining and widespread social change. All soccer-related activities delivered within the programmes focuses on peace education and community activism, in order to create a self-sustaining conflict mitigation movement.[26] The current research focused on the first phase of the project, the eight-month training stage which is the most intensive and long phase of the project, due to the understanding that the training phase is crucial for the successful of the whole project as well as due to the accessibility of the participants to the research during this stage.

Methodology

Participants

There were 48 participants in the second year of Mifalot's 'United Soccer for Peace' soccer coaches certification course. Approximately, 95% of all the participants who took part in the programme during 2013 were interviewed for this research. The participants attended three groups in different parts of Israel. In the north, (Afula) 18 male participants (10 Jewish and 8 Arab) were interviewed. In the centre of Israel (Raa'nna), a group of 20 participants was interviewed, all of them Jews, 15 women and 5 men. In the south the group consisted of 10 Jewish men. Another group of 15 participants that consisted of 14 men and 1 woman, 8 Jewish and 7 Arabs were interviewed. This group took part in the same project in the year 2012. All the participants were between the ages of 20–45 with some background in sports.

Procedure and materials

The research took place in two time phases. The first phase took place in December, 2012 in which the first group of participants from the south was interviewed. The interviews were conducted in Hebrew by graduate students from Ben Gurion University who were trained by the authors through a year-long course in evaluation of conflict mitigation through sports programmes. There were no problems with translation as all of the interviewees, including the Arabs, were fluent in conversational Hebrew. A manual to support the delivery procedure for the interview was developed by the authors and the students, and the interviewers followed this manual. The questions that were asked were focused on getting to know the participants, why they joined the project, how they felt about the 'other', how the course affected their feelings toward the 'other' and suggestions for improving the course. The interviewers were instructed to add any questions if needed for clarification. The interviews took place towards the end of the eight-month training, so the participants related to the whole training phase.

The second time phase was one year later and again the interviews were conducted by graduate students who were trained in interviewing techniques in a graduate course taught by the authors. This time the BGU students interviewed three groups, in the north (Afula), centre (Raanna) and south (Beer Sheva). In the second year, some questions were added to the manual, as a result of information received from Mifalot staff that many Arab participants left the project. The additional items focused on attempting to understand the relationship between the Jewish and Arab participants, why the Arab participants left the course, and how the course could be improved. The interviews took between 20 and 60 min, and were fully transcribed.

Data analysis

A thematic approach[27] was used in order to analyse the material. In the first phase of the analysis, the graduate students worked in small groups (2–4) and with the supervision of the researchers traced the main themes that emerged out of the interviews. In the second phase, each small group presented its themes in front of the whole group (about 20 graduate students) and the group discussed the materials. In parallel to the students work, the authors also conducted an analysis of the interviews. At the last stage of the analysis, the authors compared their analysis with the students' analysis. The themes that appeared stable in all the analysis processes are the ones, which are presented here. In order to demonstrate our results, we used quotes from the interviews.

Results

Advantages and challenges of this project in the area of group relations and peace education

Attitudes of Jews and Arabs towards each other

Generally, Jewish and Arab participants from all groups expressed positive attitudes towards each other. They expressed willingness to learn and practice together and strengthen the argument that 'people are people'. For example, Moti[28] (Jewish-north) said: 'the atmosphere in the course is very good, Jews and Arabs, we help each other, support each other'. Muhamad (Arab-North) said: 'Jewish, Arab it does not matter, we work together and feel very good together'. However, beyond the mutual general statements of both Jewish and Arab participants that the relationship between them during the training was good, when examining the interviews more carefully a much more complex picture emerged.

The 'collective' perception of Jews and Arabs

Some of the Arab Bedouin participants who live in the south of Israel expressed their wish to change the negative stereotype that Jews who live in the south have towards Arab Bedouins. For example, Salem said:

> I would like to change the way the Jews think about us, Bedouins. People (Jews) think that all Bedouins are bad, are thieves, but this is not true, on the contrary, there are many good people, people who can change things and improve the relationships between Jews and Bedouins.

The relationship between Jews and Arabs within the project

Some participants described the good atmosphere that exists during the trainings between members of the two groups. For example, Leor (Jewish) said: 'We sit and talk, during the break we tell jokes, good atmosphere', whilst another Arab interviewee said: 'We are having fun and learning together, lots of jokes, good time'. However, some interviewees, both Jews and Arabs, suggested that during the training course the relationship between them is good but there is no social connection outside the trainings. For example, Ronen (Jewish) said laughing: 'We are having fun together during the trainings but we did not became friends, it is not the case, I will not phone them and go to eat in their homes', another Arab participant added: 'During the training we collaborate and there is a good atmosphere, but at the end of the training we shake hands and go home ... no more then this'.

Changes in attitudes as a result of the project

Most of the participants claimed that their attitudes towards each other's group did not change due to the project. Many said that they came to the project with good attitudes towards the other side so there was not much to change. However, a few participants claimed that there were some changes in their attitude, following the project. For example, Samir (Arab-North) suggested:

> At the beginning, I was not sure if I will connect to the group, but then when I got to know the people, my attitude changes, I became more open ... we know that there are racist people in both communities, but when you meet the people themselves, get to know them personally then you understand that not all Jews are racists ...

Some of the Jewish participants in the mixed groups stressed the new knowledge they gained as a result of meeting and collaborating with the Arab participants. They learned about the Arab's culture, their holidays, music, food and learned to respect each other's culture. For example Shai (Jewish-Jerusalem) said: 'We learned about each other culture, different kinds of food, religious holidays ... we respected each other's holidays and we cancelled the trainings when the day falls on a holiday, and then we completed the missing material together'.

Motives for participation in the project

All of the participants said that they love sport and want to get a professional coaching certificate. For most of them, Jews and Arabs, the project served as a way to enhance their professional skills. Some acted as coaches in their communities but needed the diploma in order to continue, others claim that they love children and sport, and want to became a professional sport coaches. Only a few participants mentioned the peace education goals as a motive to take part in the project. Most of the participants, but not all, were aware of the goals of the project in the area of peace education, but did not pay much attention to it. For them it was a small additional part of the main aim, becoming a professional soccer coach. Some were positive about the fact that Jews and Arabs learn together in the project, others were indifferent, but no one rejected the idea.

Some participants, mainly Arabs but also some Jews, suggested that through their participation in the project, they would like to contribute to their communities. They stressed their role as social activists. For example, one Arab Bedouin young woman from the south, Samira, stated that her aim in participating in this project is: 'to open the world of football to Arab-Bedouin women. Another Arab Bedouin man from the south', Auda, suggested that he wants to develop professional sport among the children in his village. He said: 'our children like sport, and they are good soccer players so I can help them, it is my responsibility'. An Arab from the north, Rajib, stated that: 'I would love to work in Mifalot as a coach and to enhance projects of coexistence between Jews and Palestinian Arabs'. Hassan, a Bedouin participant from the south stated that: 'what brought me to this project is the issue of peace education, I would like to teach our children how to connect with Jewish children through sport'. One Jewish participant, a woman from the centre, Einat, claimed that she is willing to coach a group of Arab women in their town as a way to enhance sports and coexistence: 'I will happily coach a group of Arab women, I can teach them the game and then they can join the project and become coaches as well'.

Peace education contents and dynamics

The interviewees hardly mentioned peace education contents, and mainly discussed the exams which contained sports related professional contents. However, when asked about a meaningful experience during the year of the training, many related to the two-day seminar that was dedicated to peace education. For them, both Jewish and Arabs, the seminar was a place to get to know each other from a more personal perspective, as well as to collaborate beyond simply sporting activities. For example, Nir (Jewish-South) said: 'The seminar was very meaningful, we got to know each other more personally, we worked together as groups with no differences between Jews and Arabs, people were open minded and supportive and we also had fun in the evening'. David (Jewish-South) suggested that during this two days seminar Jews and Arabs felt united: 'There was this joint seminar for two days learning about peace education and it was fun, we were united, not two groups, Jews and Arabs, but one group, together, it was a great experience for me because we worked as one entity'. Hassan (Bedouin-south) added: 'It was more personal, we spoke about each other, not only soccer, it was meaningful for me'. Another Arab participant, Samir from the north, claimed that he learned from the seminar that: 'It is not about winning or losing, it is about working together as a group'.

Technical and organizational difficulties which are related to minority issues

Addressing the project in general, some organizational difficulties, which are related to the relationship between majority and minority groups, emerged. *Location of the training*: All four groups were trained in facilities that were located in Jewish cities. The reason was that the sport facilities are more advanced in those cities then in the neighbouring Arab cities and town. However, this situation forced the Arab participants to travel away from their homes and increased their feelings of being a minority. *Language of teaching*: The training was divided into field training and formal studies, which took place in the class. All the participants had to go through written exams in order to get their diploma. However, all the training was conducted in Hebrew. Using Hebrew as the only teaching language made it difficult for some of the Arab participants. *Payment for the training*: The Arab participants did not pay for the project but the Jewish participants had to pay. Only a few interviewees related to this topic, but the ones who did, which were Jewish claimed that there should be equality between all the participants.

Why did many Arab participants leave the project in its early stages?

Out of the four groups of coaches that were interviewed, which started the training as mixed groups of Jews and Arabs, only two groups remained mixed groups until the end of the training with more or less equal number of Arab and Jewish participants who started and finished the programme. These groups were male groups, except for one Bedouin young woman who remained in the southern group. In the other two groups all the Arab participants left after a few training meetings. Since the interviews took place towards the end of the eight-month training period, it was not possible to locate the Arab participants who left many months before the interviews took place and to ask them personally why they left the project, but due to the importance of the question we could and did ask the remaining Jewish participants to help us understand why the Arabs left the project. The answers varied. Some of the Jewish participants said that they truly do not know why the Arabs left the course, Dan said: 'they just left, no one spoke about it and we did not ask, we continued the training with Jews only'. Rachel added: 'I really do not know why they left, they were here for 2–3 meetings and then they disappeared and the group was so big, anyway ...' When asked if anyone tried to locate the Arab participants who left to ask them for their reasons of leaving the answers were not clear. Some Jewish participants suggested that since they left the training at the beginning, no contact was established so they did not phone and ask them. Others said that they did not have their telephone numbers or were not interested. The overall message was that no one (from the participants or \and the staff) did anything to understand why they left or\and try to make them come back to the project.

However, analysing all the data the following picture emerged. It was suggested that the orientation of most of the recruited Arab participants did not fit the project, for example, 'they were not connected to sport' or 'they did not know the game', 'you must have some background in order to get into a professional course like

theoretical basis for attempting conflict mitigation through sports. This study, through field research, actually examined the effects of a sports development programme on the attitudes of its participants and showed that indeed, a sports development programme can make significant contributions to conflict mitigation. Mifalot's 'United Soccer for Peace' programme, with its focus on the training phase, had achievements as well as challenges and aspects that can be improved.

The last part of this paper is devoted to suggestions for improving this project. Limitations of the current research included the fact that it was focused on one phase of the whole project as well as that all the interviewers were Jewish who spoke Hebrew, while interviewees were Arabs and Jews. Moreover, it would be beneficial to try and locate the Arab participants who left and interview them as well. However, a great deal of knowledge was gained from the in depth interviews, knowledge that can shed light and contribute to this programme as well as to future ones.

What can be done to improve this project and similar projects like this in the future?

Structural recommendations

Better recruitment is needed in order to get the right people to the project that will be committed to finishing the course. It is important to have more or less the same-age groups and a required physical abilities and some professional background. All the participants should pay a similar small fee or at least a deposit in order to feel committed to complete the programme. Further, it is most important to conduct the training in both Jewish and Arab cities\town, so participants who live in either place will feel integrated into the programme. An example of a successful programme that applies this concept is a folk dance programme conducted with Dr. Levi Bar-Gil in a Bedouin village near Dimona with women ages 25–55. The women meet once a week to learn new dances set to music that they have selected. One might think that a dance programme with Bedouin women led by a Jewish Israeli man would not be successful, but quite the opposite is true. The programme continues to grow in popularity and about 40 women participate each week in these dance sessions. It is recommended to recruit two trainers for each group, Jewish and Arab to train the group, so both groups will have a trainer that speaks their language and understand their culture needs and constraints. Moreover, the training should take place both in Hebrew and Arabic. The academic material should be translated into Arabic, so both Arabs and Jews will have equal accessibility to the written materials. It is also recommended to conduct the exams in both languages in order to have equal chances to pass the exams. Due to cultural differences between Jews and Muslims, it is recommended to separate between men and women and offer two separate training courses for men and women separately.

Interpersonal and dynamics recommendations

It appears very important to make a declaration of intent. Indeed, the aim of the programme in the field of peace education should be presented very clearly to the participants, during the recruitment phase but also during the training phase. Programme facilitators need better training in peace education and recreation leadership principles so that the coaches will have these skills. The leaders should enhance personal relationships between the participants during the trainings. This can be done by 'warming up' games that foster interpersonal relationships, creating some free space for open communication, organizing social activities outside the training schedule. Both professional trainers as well as programme facilitators should assist the Arabs more and help them with the course more, making sure they feel comfortable with the course material as well as socially. In case of dropouts, there should be a fast response to inquire about the reasons for dropping out and to explore options for returning to the training. Due consideration should be provided for creating more space for collaboration between Arabs and Jews – encourage potential cooperation between Jews and Arabs in the group in the training by creating mutual interest and joint assignments. Finally, it is recommended to integrate more peace education content in the trainings that can be taught academically in the class (peace education values, models, tools). It is important not to separate the seminar from the every week trainings but to try and integrate the content there were taught in the seminar during the training time and in the future as trainers with children. A key long-term focus of the programme is health and well-being. Future programmes should endeavour to collect further research on the impact of the Mifalot programme on short- and long-term health and well-being. Implementing these recommendations would enhance Mifalot's 'United Soccer for Peace' programme as well as other programmes in Israel and in other conflict areas, which attempt to use sport as a tool for conflict mitigation and health improvement

Additional remarks by the authors

ML and YG: It is July 2014 and many rockets and missiles have been fired at Israel from Gaza in the last 11 days. Israel has been bombing the terrorist infrastructure in Gaza to try to stop the rocket attacks. A skeptic might say that this war is an indication that programmes like 'United Soccer for Peace' do not work. On the contrary, it shows that these programmes are more important than ever and need to expand to reach more people. Acts of violence can lead to more hatred which leads to more violence which leads to more hatred and things can spiral out of control. Here in Tel Aviv during this crisis, with occasional 'red alert' sirens forcing us to run for shelter, it would be easy to look to the source of the rocket fire and feel a general hatred toward Arabs. However, this is not the case at all for me. Through my involvement with the Mifalot programmes I know that it would be wrong to feel that way and I believe that others involved in Mifalot programmes are like me and have a greater sense of the bigger picture and will not resort to hatred and violence even in difficult times such as these. In a conclusion, the 'United Soccer for Peace' programme and similar efforts are more important now than ever before.

TLH: As an Israeli, who lives in the south of Israel and teaches Peace education at the university, I often hear from my graduate students' criticism about the naivety and unusefulness of peace programmes. My answer to them and to myself is that 'if we manage to change one person's attitude and\or behavior through these programmes, we achieve one small step towards peace'. I believe that through sports and programmes like the 'United Soccer for Peace', many small steps towards peace are achieved.

Acknowledgements
We would like to thank Mifalot for allowing us to conduct this research. We would like to thank all our graduate students who helped us in gathering the information for this research.

Disclosure statement

No potential conflict of interest was reported by the authors.

Notes

1. Bairner, 'Sport, Ireland, and Identity', 222; Ford, 'Basketball in Sustainable Peacebuilding', 723; Lidor and Blumenstein, 'Players from Conflicting Cultures', 229; Malcolm, 'Cricket, Violence, and Conflict', 215; Rookwood, 'Soccer for Peace Development', 474; Rookwood, 'Sport Initiative in Russia', 230; Schinke et al., 'Toward Trust and Partnership', 201; Schulenkorf, 'Sports Events and Reconciliation', 201; Schulenkorf and Sugden, 'Sport Development and Peace', 255; Schulenkorf, Sugden, and Burdsey, 'Sport as Contested Terrain', 275; Skille, 'Conventions of Sports Clubs', 245; Sugden, 2006, Sugden, 'Football for Peace?' 45; 2010; Tuohey and Cognate, 'Peace Players International', 55.
2. Leitner, Galily, and Shimon, 'Sports Programmes on Attitudes', 237; Schulenkorf, Sugden, and Burdsey, 'Sport as Contested Terrain', 375.
3. Schulenkorf and Sugden, 'Sport Development and Peace', 239; Leitner, Galily, and Shimon, 'Sports Programs on Attitudes', 238.
4. Allport, *The Nature of Prejudice*, 21.
5. Kidd, 'Sport Development and Peace', 375.
6. Tuohey and Cognate, 'Peace Players International', 51.
7. Ibid., 52.
8. Levermore, 'Sport Engine of Development?' 185.
9. Merton, 'Empirical Research on Sociology', 509; Parsons, *The Social System*, 22.
10. Sugden's 2006; Sugden, 'Football for Peace?' 45; 2010.
11. Schulenkorf, 'Sports Events and Reconciliation', 277.
12. Rookwood, 'Sport Initiative in Russia', 231.
13. Galily, 'Sport, Politics and Society in Israel', 517.
14. Leitner and Leitner, *Israeli Life and Leisure*, 54; Seginer and Mahajna, 'Beliefs about Women's Roles', 124.
15. Smooha, *Arab–Jewish Relations in Israel*, 44.
16. Zureik and Moughrabi, *Public Opinion, Palestine Question*, 88.
17. Smooha, Arabs, Jews in Israel, 101.
18. Tajfel and Turner, 'SI Theory Intergroup Behavior', 13.
19. Allport, *The Nature of Prejudice*, 51.
20. Amir, 'Prejudice and Ethnic Relations', 247; Jackson, 'Contact Theory of Hostility', 48; Maoz, 'Power Relations in Encounters', 45.
21. Amir, 'Prejudice and Ethnic Relations', 250; Jackson, 'Contact Theory of Hostility', 48; Maoz, 'Power Relations in Encounters', 45.
22. Schulenkorf, Sugden, and Burdsey, 'Sport as Contested Terrain', 277.
23. Schulenkorf and Sugden, 'Sport Development and Peace', 240.
24. Leitner, Galily, and Shimon, 'Sports Programs on Attitudes', 240.
25. Ibid.
26. Kamil, *United Soccer for Peace*, 27.
27. Lieblich, Tuval-Mashiach, and Zilber, *Narrative Research*, 37; Skedi, 'Conventions of Sports Clubs', 44.
28. All names are pseudo names.
29. Sugden 2006; Sugden, 'Football for Peace?' 48; 2010.
30. Schulenkorf, 'Sports Events and Reconciliation', 47.
31. Leitner, Galily, and Shimon, 'Sports Programs on Attitudes', 242.
32. Allport, *The Nature of Prejudice*, 59.
33. Amir, 'Prejudice and Ethnic Relations', 251; Maoz, 'Power Relations in Encounters', 260.
34. Ram, 'Post-Zionism in Global Age', 225.
35. Seginer and Mahajna, 'Beliefs about Women's Roles', 125; Smooha, *Arab–Jewish Relations in Israel*, 33.
36. Kamil, *United Soccer for Peace*, 78.

37. Schulenkorf and Sugden, 'Sport Development and Peace', 256.
38. Allport, *The Nature of Prejudice*, 62.
39. Maoz, 2004.
40. Maoz, 2002; Maoz, 'Evaluating Intergroup Encounter Interventions', 262; Suleiman, 'Planned encounters between Israelis', 325.
41. Seginer and Mahajna, 'Beliefs about Women's Roles', 128; Smooha, *Arab–Jewish relations in Israel*, 130.
42. Seginer and Mahajna, 'Beliefs about Women's Roles', 128.
43. Maoz, 'Evaluating Intergroup Encounter Interventions', 263; Suleiman, 'Planned Encounters between Israelis', 326.
44. Rookwood, 'Sport Initiative in Russia', 230.
45. Levermore, 'Sport Engine of Development?' 188; Kidd, 'Sport Development and Peace', 371; Rookwood, 'Soccer for Peace Development', 231; Sugden, 'Critical Left-realism and Sport Interventions in Divided Societies' 2010.

References

Allport, G.W. *The Nature of Prejudice*. Reading, MA: Addison-Wesley, 1954.
Amir, Y. 'The Role of Intergroup Contact in Change of Prejudice and Ethnic Relations'. In *Towards the Elimination of Racism*, ed. P.A. Katz, 245–308. New York: Pergamon, 1976.
Bairner, A. 'Sport, the Northern Ireland Peace Process, and the Politics of Identity'. *Journal of Aggression, Conflict and Peace Research* 5, no. 4 (2013): 220–9.
Ford, C. 'Peace and Hoops: Basketball as a Role Player in Sustainable Peacebuilding'. *Willamette Law Review* 42 (2006): 723–4.
Gal, R. *Summary of 1994 Attitudinal Research*. ZichronYaacov: The Carmel Institute, 1996, March 1.
Galily, Y. 'Sport, Politics and Society in Israel: The First Fifty-five Years'. *Israel Affairs* 13, no. 3 (2007): 515–28.
Galily, Y., M.J. Leitner, and P. Shimion. 'The Effects of Three Israeli Sports Programs on Attitudes of Arabs and Jews toward One Another'. *Journal of Aggression, Conflict and Peace Research* 5, no. 4 (2013): 243–58.
Jackson, J.W. 'Contact Theory of Intergroup Hostility: A Review and Evaluation of the Theoretical and Empirical Literature'. *International Journal of Group Tensions* 23 (1993): 43–65.
Kamil, N. *Information about the United Soccer for Peace Coaches Training*. Tel Aviv: Mifalot, 2012.
Kidd, B. 'A New Social Movement: Sport for Development and Peace'. *Sport in Society* 11, no. 4 (2008): 370–80.
Leitner, M.J., Y. Galily, and P. Shimon. 'The Effects of Peres Center for Peace Sports Programs on the Attitudes of Arab and Jewish Israeli Youth'. *Leadership and Policy Quarterly* 1, no. 2 (2012): 109–21.
Leitner, M.J., Y. Galily, and P. Shimon. 'A Two-year Study on the Effects of the Friendship Games on Attitudes towards Arabs and Jews'. *World Leisure Journal* 56, no. 3 (2014): 236–52.
Leitner, M.J., and S.F. Leitner, eds. *Israeli Life and Leisure in the 21st Century*. Urbana, IL: Sagamore, 2014.
Levermore, R. 'Sport a New Engine of Development?' *Progress in Development Studies* 8, no. 2 (2008): 183–90.
Lidor, R., and B. Blumenstein. 'Working with Adolescent Soccer and Basketball Players from Conflicting Cultures – A Three-dimensional Consultation Approach'. *Journal of Sport and Social Issues* 35, no. 3 (2011): 229–45.
Lieblich, A., R. Tuval, and T. Zilber. *Narrative Research: Reading, Analysis, and Interpretation*. Thousand Oaks, CA: Sage, 1998.
Malcolm, D. 'Cricket, Violence and Social Conflict: An Eliasian Examination'. *Journal of Aggression, Conflict and Peace Research* 5, no. 4 (2013): 211–9.
Maoz, I. 'Power Relations in Intergroup Encounters: A Case Study of Jewish–Arab Encounters in Israel'. *International Journal of Intercultural Relations* 24, no. 2 (2000): 259–77.

Maoz, I. 'Coexistence is in the Eye of the Beholder: Evaluating Intergroup Encounter Interventions between Jews and Arabs in Israel'. *Journal of Social Issues* 60, no. 2 (2004): 437–52.

Merton, R. 'The Bearing of Empirical Research upon the Development of Social Theory'. *American Sociological Review* 13 (1948): 505–15.

Parsons, T. *The Social System*. Glencoe, IL: Free Press, 1951.

Ram, U. 'The Promised Land of Business Opportunities: Liberal Post-Zionism in the Global Age'. In *The New Israel*, ed. G. Shafir and Y. Peled, 217–40. Boulder, CO: Westview Press, 2000.

Rookwood, J. 'Soccer for Peace and Social Development'. *Peace Review* 20 (2008): 471–9.

Rookwood, J. 'Building from Beslan: Examining and NGO Community Sport Initiative in Russia and Its Capacity to Promote Peace amongst Victims of Terrorism'. *Journal of Aggression, Conflict and Peace Research* 5, no. 4 (2013): 230–42.

Schinke, R.J., K.R. McGannon, J. Watson, and R. Busanich. 'Moving toward Trust and Partnership: An Example of Sport-related Community-based Participatory Action Research with Aboriginal People and Mainstream Academics'. *Journal of Aggression, Conflict and Peace Research* 5, no. 4 (2013): 201–10.

Schulenkorf, N. 'Sport Events and Ethnic Reconciliation: Attempting to Create Social Change between Sinhalese, Tamil, and Muslim Sportspeople in War Torn Sri Lanka'. *International Review for the Sociology of Sport* 45, no. 3 (2010): 273–94.

Schulenkorf, N., and J. Sugden. 'Sport for Development and Peace in Divided Societies: Cooperating for Inter-community Empowerment in Israel'. *European Journal for Sport and Society* 8, no. 4 (2011): 235–56.

Schulenkorf, N., J. Sugden, and D. Burdsey. 'Sport for Development and Peace as Contested Terrain: Place, Community, Ownership'. *International Journal of Sport Policy and Politics* 6 (2014): 371–87. doi:10.1080/19406940.2013.825875.

Seginer, R., and S. Mahajna. 'How the Future Orientation of Traditional Israeli Palestinian Girls Links Beliefs about Women's Roles and Academic Achievement'. *Psychology of Women Quarterly* 28 (2004): 122–35.

Skille, E. 'The Conventions of Sport Clubs: Enabling and Constraining the Implementation of Social Goods through Sport'. *Sport, Education and Society* 16, no. 2 (2011): 241–53.

Smooha, S. *Arabs and Jews in Israel: Volume 1*. Boulder, CO.: Westview Press, 1989.

Smooha, S. *Arab–Jewish Relations in Israel: Alienation and Rapprochement*. Peaceworks No. 67. Washington, DC: The United States Institute of Peace, 2010.

Sugden, J. 'The Challenge of Using a Values-based Approach to Coaching Sport and Community Relations in Multi-cultural Settings: The Case of Football for Peace (F4P) in Israel'. *European Journal for Sport and Society* 3, no. 1 (2006): 7–27.

Sugden, J. 'Sport and Community Relations in Northern Ireland and Israel'. In *Sport and the Irish: Histories, Identities, Issues, Sport and the Irish: Histories, Identities, Issues*, ed. A. Bairner, 251f. Dublin: University College Dublin Press, 2006.

Sugden, J. 'Teaching and Playing Sport for Conflict Resolution and Co-existence in Israel'. *International Review for the Sociology of Sport* 41, no. 2 (2006): 221–40.

Sugden, J. 'Anyone for Football for Peace? The Challenges of Using Sport in the Service of Co-existence in Israel'. *Soccer & Society* 9, no. 3 (2008): 405–15.

Sugden, J. 'Between Idealism and Fatalism: Critical Realism, Sport and Social Intervention'. In *Fostering Peace through Cultural Initiatives. From the Roundtable on Conflict and Culture*, ed. JRIPEC, 33–53. London: The Japan Foundation, 2010.

Sugden, J. 'Critical Left-realism and Sport Interventions in Divided Societies'. *International Review for the Sociology of Sport* 45 (2010): 258–72.

Suleiman, R. 'Planned Encounters between Jewish and Palestinian Israelis: A Social-psychological Perspective'. *Journal of Social Issues* 60, no. 2 (2004): 323–37.

Tajfel, H., and J. Turner. 'The Social Identity Theory of Intergroup Behavior'. In *Psychology of Intergroup Relations*, ed. S. Worchel and W. Austin, 7–24. Chicago, IL: Nelson-Hall, 1986.

Tuohey, B., and B. Cognato. 'PeacePlayers International: A Case Study on the Use of Sport as a Tool for Conflict Transformation'. *SAIS Review* 31, no. 1 (2011): 51–63.

Zureik, E., and F. Moughrabi. *Public Opinion and the Palestine Question*. New York: St. Martin Press, 1987.

The pursuit of lifelong participation: the role of professional football clubs in the delivery of physical education and school sport in England

Daniel Parnell[a,1], Sarah Buxton[b], Des Hewitt[c], Matthew J. Reeves[d], Ed Cope[e] and Richard Bailey[f]

[a]Carnegie Faculty, Centre for Active Lifestyles, Leeds Beckett University, Leeds, UK; [b]Department of Education, University of Derby, Derby, UK; [c]Centre for Professional Education, University of Warwick, Coventry, UK; [d]School of Education, Leisure & Sport Studies, Liverpool John Moores University, IM Marsh Campus, Liverpool, UK; [e]Sports Coaching, Sheffield Hallam, Sheffield, UK; [f]International Council of Sport Science and Physical Education, Berlin, Germany

Physical Education and School Sport (PESS) offers a key vehicle to support the development of lifelong participation in children and young people. At a time of government cuts and the emergence of external providers, including professional football clubs, it is pertinent to explore current practice. This research set out to explore the delivery, and partnerships involved within the School Sports Premium, particularly the relationship between the community arms and registered charities of professional football clubs and schools to deliver PESS. Semi-structured interviews with community managers from football community programmes and head teachers revealed two key themes; partnership working and the role of the community coach. Findings suggest the need to develop the scope of the partnership and to build methods of evaluation to understand the impact of the coaches' practice in schools. Further evaluation of the partnerships between professional football clubs and schools would bring an increased understanding of the effectiveness and impact of the partnerships, in order to improve practice and the subsequent effectiveness of PESS, in terms of its contribution towards lifelong participation for children and young people.

Introduction

Physical Education and School Sport (PESS) has been documented as a complex and politicized context.[1] It is fair to summarize PESS England, in terms of subject marginalization, resource deficit and policy indifference. PESS, in particularly, has been expected to achieve multiple outcomes by a range of stakeholders,[2] including the promotion of physical activity (PA), which is a major consideration for the National Institute for Health and Care Excellence (NICE)[3] in order to support lifelong participation. In the post Olympic era, and the funding cuts and subsequent dismantling of School Sports Partnership Programme, which was previously spearheaded by the Youth Sport Trust (YST).

---

[1]Current affiliation: Faculty of Business and Law, Business in Sport, Centre for Business and Society, Business School, Manchester Metropolitan University, UK.

The new coalition government announced a new investment in PESS through the PE and Sport Premium for primary schools. This involved the distribution of over £450 million directly to primary school head teachers to improve PESS between 2013 and 2016. This investment has resulted in the re-emergence and upsurge of a new type of external provider after a short, but difficult year before the announcement of the PE and Sport premium. The decentralization of decision-making on this investment to head teachers has seen a range of willing external providers that include small businesses, charities, social entrepreneurs and professional football clubs. These organizations compete for this PESS funding. To our knowledge there is very little known and even less research as to the role of external providers working in PESS, especially professional football clubs. This research set out to explore the delivery and partnerships involved within the current PESS landscape.

Background

The promotion of PA is a major Public Health concern given the mounting evidence of its importance in increasing longevity and quality of life.[4] Many non-communicable diseases, including cardiovascular disease, obesity and high blood pressure, track from childhood through to adulthood.[5] Taking into account that one in three to five children in the Western world is overweight or obese,[6] promoting PA during childhood is firmly on the Public Health agenda. The case for the promotion of PA has been further enhanced by the developing empirical base relating it to a host of positive non-physical-health outcomes, including improved cognitive functioning, strengthened self-esteem and increased employability.[7] PESS has been seen as a means to facilitate PA opportunities for children to develop lifelong participation.

Within England, the NICE offers guidance for promoting PA for children and young people.[8] This includes 15 recommendations, all of which offer resonance for schools. Through PESS and a variety of incidental opportunities during the school period, the school setting can play a major contributing role in children and young people's PA.[9] PE, in particular, has long been expected to realize multiple aims. In addition to its role as a key societal vehicle for the promotion of health-enhancing PA, it is also expected to be the platform for the teaching of fundamental movement skills, encourage voluntary sports engagement and contribute to talent development.[10] The challenges faced by those leading and delivering PE during the latter decades of the twentieth century have been well documented, and it is fair to summarize the results in England in terms of subject marginalization, resource deficit and policy indifference.[11] However, the growing political interest in sport, echoed in education, notably around the potential of PESS to contribute to broader political policy objectives has been substantial. Consequently, by 2002, the New Labour government decided to make PESS one of its policy priorities. The launch of the national PESS and Club Links (PESSCL) strategy in 2002 represented a major political and financial commitment by the Labour government to the creation of a ground-breaking infrastructure for PESS. Its rationale was that all children, whatever their circumstances or abilities, should be able to participate in and enjoy PESS.[12]

A major development and investment in PESS was through the national/local strategic pooling of resources, through Specialist Sports Colleges and School Sports Coordinators with School Sport Partnerships (SSPs), under the banner of PESSCL (later rebranded as PESS for Young People – PESSYP). It is worth offering some contextualization to the importance of specialist colleges. Nationally there are specialist colleges for technology, languages, etc., therefore for sport to be recognized as an important curriculum subject it also became an option for specialist school status. The position of the YST within the development of PESS in England is highly significant, and worth noting. Whilst it was formally a charity, under the New Labour government it acquired a status more akin to a government department, as can be seen by its inclusion alongside actual departments in documents like the DCMS' Playing to Win.[13] A key target of the PESSCL was to enhance the sporting opportunities for young people.[14]

These key movements, helped along by the growing political and popular interest in sport, helped inform the bid for London 2012, an Olympic Games that would – it was claimed – act as a vehicle to endorse and promote sports participation for all social groups, particularly children and young people.[15] On securing the bid for the Olympic Games, PSA Target 22 aimed to deliver a successful Olympic and Paralympic Games with a sustainable 'legacy' and to get more young people taking part in PE and sport.[16] The candidate file asserted a commitment to a legacy for the Games to capture the long-term benefits of the Games including its promise to inspire a generation of young people in participation and sport, and to get more children and young people taking part in high quality PESS.[17]

The election of a new Coalition Government in 2010, made up of right-leaning Conservatives and left-leaning Liberal Democrats saw an abrupt end to many of these developments for PESS. This was part of the government's Comprehensive Spending Review enacted in 2010 to be achieved by 2014. The combination of a global economic downturn and English Treasury and Education departments adhering to broadly neo-liberal economics meant that the extravagantly funded PESSCL and PESSYP suite of programmes were judged as no longer tenable.[18] In October 2010, the new Secretary of State for Education Michael Gove wrote an open letter to Sue Campbell, the Chair of the YST, informing her that his department would no longer be providing ring-fenced funding for SSPs, and would end the £162 million PESSYP funding in order to give schools the time and freedom to focus on providing competitive sport.[19]

In many ways, the new schools competition framework was really a repackaging of elements of school games events that were part of PESSCL and PESSYP. However, the explicit focus on competitive events, which can only have a sustained impact on a minority of the school population, led some to question their long-term benefit.[20] A new youth sport policy document, Creating a sporting habit for life: a new youth sport strategy, suggested that a new approach for Britain is needed, which would be a more rigorous and targeted way of thinking that focuses on results within grassroots sport and school-club links.[21]

> Improving links between schools and community sports clubs – we will work with sports such as Football, Cricket, Rugby Union, Rugby League and Tennis to establish at least 6000 partnerships between schools and local sports clubs by 2017 – making it easier for young people to continue playing sport once they leave education. (4)[22]

Around this time, the Government announced the PE and Sport Premium for primary schools, and its intention to distribute over £450 million directly allocated to primary school head-teachers to improve PESS in primary schools between 2013 and 2016. This was a shift in focus from central management, to a competitive environment of less legislation and decentralized, local decision-making. The change in the funding landscape was by accompanying changes in delivery and curriculum. The generous investment that accompanied PESSCL/PESSYP fostered the emergence of a new type of external provider. The decentralized funding pattern that replaced these schemes, along with the availability of the PE and Sport Premium for primary schools, supported this development further. The result was that primary school PESS in England became taught by an unprecedented range of deliverers, including small businesses, charities, social entrepreneurs and professional sports clubs. Within this context, football emerged as a key agent within schools. This was magnified further when, in 2014, the English Premier League announced the launch of substantial investment in a 3-year programme of support and delivery of PESS in Primary School.[23]

Given the public interest and mass youth appeal of football, it is hardly surprising that it has been seen as a key vehicle to deliver on social agendas.[24] Indeed, football has a long history of involvement in government-supported community programmes.[25] Clubs played key roles in their local areas, helping to reinforce a sense of place and local identity. In this regard, football and community have become closely linked. The development of the notion of 'community institutions' took shape in the form of the national Football in the Community (FitC) programme in the 1970s.[26]

Professional football clubs have developed a range of community-based, social partnerships, including those with local authorities and schools.[27] Community programmes covered a range of issues and agendas, from health improvement for men,[28] women,[29] families,[30] older adults,[31] social engagement, inclusion and disability,[32] anti-social behaviour,[33] education and literacy. The recent Premier League School Sport Programme has extended to engagement directly into lessons and to the support of teacher professional development.[34] Such community-oriented work (or corporate social responsibility) has seen a shift from being a perceived philanthropic pursuit to a strategic management tool, which is seen as essential to engaging and maintaining supporters and sponsors, and to ensure more effective relations with local authorities.[35] Research and evaluation is fundamental for gauging effectiveness,[36] yet there remains very little research of the role of professional football clubs community programmes delivering PESS.[37] Conducting research and evaluation can contribute to the development of effective partnership working.[38]

Given the lack of understanding on the implementation of PESS for young people and its potential for the development of lifelong participation, this research set out to explore the delivery and partnerships involved within PESS between schools and professional football clubs, specifically delivering on the School Sports Premium. Offering considerations to inform policy development and future practice across education, school sport, PE and professional football clubs at a local and national level. To our knowledge there is very little is known and even less research the role of external providers working in PESS, especially professional football clubs. This research set out to explore the delivery and partnerships involved within the current PESS landscape between professional football clubs and schools.

Methods

Research context

This study was undertaken in schools and professional football clubs in the East and West Midlands of England. Specifically, the participants involved representatives from the counties of Derbyshire, Leicestershire and Staffordshire. Derbyshire, at the time of writing, had 303 primary schools delivering education for children up to the age of 11 years. Leicestershire had 201 primary schools and Staffordshire had 274 primary schools.

The primary head teachers ($n = 7$) involved in the research were recruited via established contacts. An additional interview was undertaken with a Consortium Operation Manager from a Co-operative Learning Trust (CLT). The CLT is a group of schools that work in collaboration from sharing practice to resources to maximize the potential opportunity for each respective school. CLTs are usually formed due to shared geographical proximity and philosophical approach. These participants were grouped together as head teachers ($n = 8$), who engaged in a semi-structured interview (see Table 1). This sample was chosen as it included schools that worked with a range of external PESS-based providers, including professional football clubs. These are collectively referred to as head teachers.

The professional football clubs FitC programmes involved in the research ($n = 4$) were part of the Football League competition and all participants were Heads of Community (referred to as community managers here on in). The community managers ($n = 4$) from the football clubs engaged in a semi-structured interview (see Table 2). Participating FitC programmes were established as registered charities and had an average turnover between £300,000 and £800,000. The community programmes had a range of provision in place covering a range of areas aligned with the key pillars of the Football League Trust.[39] Importantly, the community programmes were involved in the provision of curriculum-based PESS provision. Participants were recruited through the support of the Football League Trust via an introductory email inviting participation in the research. All data collection took place between April and June 2013. Ethical approval was granted via University of Derby University Ethics Committee, and all participants provided informed consent.

A semi-structured interview schedule (see Tables 1 and 2) was deductively developed using previous research on the PESS and related to PA as a guide.[40] This was supplemented to consider both previous partnership research[41] and with consideration to NICE guidance for promoting PA for children and young people.[42] The researchers had previous experience of research, management and deliver of PESS including within school managed curriculum delivery, external PESS delivery organizations and partnerships between schools and professional football clubs.

Table 1. Semi-structured interview themes for head teachers.

- Professional background
- Learning philosophies and strategies
- Views of effective teaching
- Views and experiences of PESS
- Views and experiences of partnerships

Table 2. Semi-structured interview for community managers.

- Professional background
- Personal and organizational coaching philosophy
- Views and experiences of PESS
- Perceptions of key stakeholders in PESS
- Views and experiences of schools and community football/sport partnerships

Data analysis and representation

Semi-structured interviews were recorded, each lasting approximately 45 min and were transcribed verbatim. Within the analysis, the participant's names were replaced with pseudonyms so that verbatim quotes could be assigned to respective participants. A thematic analysis approach was undertaken,[43] which included finding and extracting common themes. Authors (DP, DH, SB) each independently read through the transcripts several times and began identifying common terms and terminology across the discourses. Firstly, themes were extracted amongst all community managers, then amongst head teachers interviews. The authors then collaborated common themes between both interview sets to help locate key themes. The themes are supplemented by verbatim citations (i.e. direct quotes) to demonstrate the contextual meaning.[44] These are identified in italics and indentations within the text.

Results

The results offer an insight into the delivery and partnership contexts between professional football clubs and schools in the era of the new PE and Sport Premium for primary schools. The two key themes that were identified are partnership working and the role of the community coach.

Partnership working

The nature of this work emphasizes the importance of partnerships and working in collaboration. So, not surprisingly participants reported that the partnership was a key feature and important consideration for both the head teachers and community managers for PESS. The legacy of the SSPs was evident within the discussions, as indicated by these participant accounts:

> We have plenty of partnerships in place, many existing within schools from the schools partnership programme [*SSP*]. I'm not from an educational background, but we see that we bring a major value to schools. (Mrs Coalter – Head of Moreton Primary School)

> We used to have a school sports partnership and they were quite effective vehicle to get external bodies involved. We are in the process of trying to re-build partnerships developed during the school sports partnership times that have been lost more recently. (Mrs Brennan – Head of Wildcoates Primary School)

> There was a structure in place for the school-sport partnership, which now lost, takes away the natural progression and exit routes. (Dave – Head of Abbey Football in the Community)

It was evident that the previous structures of the SSP reached and engaged both schools and footballs clubs and other local community organizations. In its absence schools appear to have highlighted that they have shouldered some of the responsibility for developing external partnerships.

The development of these partnerships appears to have been positively influenced by the work of the SSPs. However, the community managers offered a more pragmatic understanding of partnership operations:

> If you cannot provide something yourself, then you work with a partner. It's straightforward really. Schools need sport coaches, which we provide. But for specialist sports

like gymnastics and swimming we partner with people to deliver too. It just makes sense. (Paul – Head of Parkview Football in the Community)

Evidently, some head teachers did not just frame the clubs' role in terms of filling a gap in provision, but also in terms of drawing in sport-specific expertise. Interestingly, some participants identified a void in the post-SSP era. These participants believed that the current partnerships required development with regard to the need to make more efficient changes to structures and resources supporting PESS within the SSP structure:

I think firstly, there's a gap on who is going to be that congruent in place of the school sport partnerships, obviously they have now disbanded. I was of the opinion that there was too many of them and it wasn't a great investment, but I am not convinced cutting away the entire structure is the best way. We need something or someone in that place, which has been left behind them. (Gary – Head of United Football in the Community)

Lumping resources into the responsibility of the head teacher of a school can be either a blessing or a nightmare. Head teachers can be a huge supporter of PE and sport, whilst others can be less so, which makes it difficult to develop partnerships at times. I know we would benefit from a specialist who can coordinate this new funding. (Mike – Head of Glenavon Football in the Community)

Whilst community managers identified a gap left in the absence of the SSP, there was a hope that the vast resources associated with the previous system would allow further opportunities at the discretion of the head teachers. However, the community managers, who many may assume would adopt commercial philosophies associated with professional football clubs, exhibited a more philanthropic approach to dealing with the concerns associated with the absence of the SSPs, and in turn partnership working:

There was a structure in place for the school-sports-partnerships, which now gone, has taken a natural progression and exit routes away. Which then puts more focus on us as an organisation and the past we would have probably just gone in, coached and stepped away. But ethically we now need to working with those local clubs and finding exit routes. Yes it is probably not seen as our role we are not funded to do that, but we need to look at the bigger picture and I think that we all need to do this for the good of sport across the board. (Paul – Head of Parkview Football in the Community)

This highlights the apparent removal of progression pathways and exit routes for children and young people, which created a gap in provision. In this instance, it was apparent that the football club was picking responsibility for this identified shortfall. Despite this evidence of commitment from the football clubs, the sustainability of the PE and Sport Premium for primary schools funding was a continued concern shared by all participants. Whilst concerns alluded to the potential influence of head teachers' philosophies, head teachers held their own suspicions:

You might get people trying to work in schools, to build a partnership, and they are willing to come in at a discounted rate, pay for a facility, and throw more into a deal. But you have to question, Who these guys are? Are the any good? Is this a sustainable approach? My guess is that most of the deals are too good to true. (Mrs Brennan – Head of Wildcoates Primary School)

Such comments suggest that there is little quality marks available to differentiate between external providers including professional football clubs. Moreover, many participants highlighted that the new partnerships had become reliant on (and in some cases focused on) funding:

> Funding is a major one, I mean you know the government has given us this amount of money now for schools, to bring in the coaches and have these new school partnerships with whoever we choose. But when that goes we are going to be able to sustain any of this? Its unlikely we will be able to sustain those kind of partnerships without the funding. (Mrs Coalter – Head of Moreton Primary School)

These are major concerns for any new or developing partnerships. The absence of clarity on the motivations for and philosophies within the partnership may be a result of a focus on the more tangible deliverables. Indeed, a major topic of conversations and a reoccurring key element related to partnerships was the importance of ensuring quality coaching. Moreover, participants made suggestions that quality coaching contributed to the development of strong partnerships:

> There is some real benefits for working in partnership, especially good quality coaching. (Mr Smith – Head of Townfield Primary School)

> Umm, I suppose if these partnerships are based on coaches that are really good quality coaches then its having that, then bringing that into school, because teachers see that as well. (Mrs Coalter – Head of Moreton Primary School)

> You need to make sure that whatever is happening, there is some quality assurance in place for the partnership. I think this is the big issue at the moment, which is going to be a big mine-field if you don't get it right, is the assurance that you are getting quality coaching and the partnership is going to work well. (Mike – Head of Glenavon Football in the Community)

Partnerships formed a central element in these conversations. According to some, the quality and sustainability of the partnership was the most important factor in the success of the relationship between schools and professional football clubs.

The role of the coach

Partnerships could be said to comprise an interaction of a wide range of variables, including funding, administration, leadership, values and human resources. Within the context of the partnerships being examined here, there seems little doubt that representatives of both schools and professional football clubs placed a considerable importance on the role of the coach. Perhaps this is not surprising, as the coach could be said to be the external face of the club. However, the coach also led the actual delivery of the programme in the schools. So, the partnership can be framed in terms of an exchange of human capital through the provision of sports coaching. In the light of this, it is not surprising that participants focused attention on this topic:

> I've seen some really good planning and preparation from the sports coaches. (Mrs McDermott – Consortium Manager of Hale Co-operative Trust)

> Qualified coaches who've been through a proper programme in order to teach sport, better able to teach that sport than teachers. (Mr Smith – Head of Townfield Primary School)

Moreover, participants from schools identified that primary teachers may exhibit limits in their practical ability in and experience of PESS. This deficiency appears to drive the perceived need for and subsequent benefits of specialist support:

> It's good to get coaches into school to teach specifics...it is quite hard for teachers unless they've done the training and have got a love for that kind of sport it's difficult for them to coach it if you like. (Mrs Coalter – Head of Moreton Primary School

> If you've got skilled coaches who have got that set and expertise they are better in my experience teaching PE to the children than most teachers. Most teachers don't have the level of coaching expertise for them to coach sports well. (Mrs Brennan – Head of Wildcoates Primary School)

> I'm also conscious a lot of teachers aren't necessarily getting to it [to deliver PESS] either. They do what they have to do, but I think whilst we would prefer coaches to come in, I would like teachers to deliver some PESS. So I think it's a balancing act. (Ms Edwards – Head of Xavier Primary School)

Experience, skills, willingness and motivation appeared to contribute to the teachers' engagement in PESS. Indeed, the value of the partnership may extend beyond a simple direct transfer of funding for coaches. There was a bigger picture and added value from the partnerships they had created. Notably, head teachers highlighted that teachers used external coaches as an opportunity to develop professionally:

> I think its almost continuing professional development for teachers to see the coaches working and to get the opportunity to have a look at that. (Ms Edwards – Head of Xavier Primary School)

> It's the idea we have coaches working alongside teachers and developing their [the teachers] coaching skills. (Mr Smith – Head of Townfield Primary School)

This continued professional development opportunity was something shared by the community managers, who alluded to a similar reciprocal learning from the coach–teacher exchanges:

> Our coaches pick-up some new ideas for good classroom behaviour management. They [coaches and teachers] give each other them ideas for curriculum and that sort of thing, but this is not a formal part of what we do, it just kind of happens. (Mike – Head of Glenavon Football in the Community)

This potential knowledge exchange did not appear to follow a coherent programme or align with any strategic or formalized intent. Participants highlighted a number of other unintended outcomes. The head teachers were keen to highlight and welcome a 'male' role model, it is clear that they also felt there is scope to broaden the role of the coach:

> We work with our local football coaches. A really important thing for us is the presence and impact of male role models coming to the school. We have very few males in the teaching staff. (Mrs Murphy – St Francis Primary School)

> So what I would always say is those coaches who will bring a lot to it need to be a lot more, they need to enter the world of the teacher and bring some of our approaches in the classroom to the gym. (Mrs Coalter – Head of Moreton Primary School)

> So to have some kind of understanding of how to teach without make it obvious you're teaching. We teachers have a lot of the time to do this, but the coaches coming in do not necessarily have this. It depends where the coaches come from that is important to say and some coaches come in and they have an awareness of the education agenda to liaise with the school to find out what they want them to do, they don't just turn up with a bag of kit and say well we are doing this today. However, some coaches lack this awareness. (Mrs Brennan – Head of Wildcoates Primary School)

These quotations suggest and reflect the schools need for male role models [not assuming all community coaches are male] and that the scope of the role of the community coach could broaden to reflect common teaching practices within a specific school context. The community managers shared some of this feeling. Moreover, they highlighted further challenges in recruiting the right kind of community coaches that could deliver a quality coaching session and also in being able to evaluate the success of their sessions:

> An important development would be for teachers to share new ideas for good classroom management behaviour with coaches, giving them ideas for curriculum and that sort of thing. (Gary – Head of United Football in the Community)

> If we put a job advert out there for a coach, people think automatically yeah it is coaching people to be better footballers, for people to be progressing into elites from grassroots into elites, but community coaches will be going into schools. In fact, our community coaches will work with one year olds to 60 years olds. (Paul – Head of Parkview Football in the Community)

> Every coach comes away from a session and they know if it's gone well. But aside from that, we haven't really got any evaluation. Although we do complete quality assurance and develop for coaches. (Jason – Head of Rovers Football in the Community)

It is clear that the partnership between the school and football club could be strengthened for more effective delivery. The role of professional development as part of capacity building within football clubs, the school and the partnership contexts appeared as an important factor that emerged. One participant highlighted the success of including professional development and capacity building within the partnership:

> Professional development is a key part of the partnership. It creates new provision and builds capacity, which for me, is the more important aspect in terms of your partnership. If you don't have that right moving forward then you are in trouble. All the schools we worked with last year have continued with us this year, because we embed capacity building into our work. (Dave – Head of Abbey Football in the Community)

Partnerships are based on the exchange of human capital by way of the provision of coaches and coaching to schools. Both head teachers and community managers highlighted the importance of high quality coaching and the unintended mutually beneficial continuing professional development opportunities.

Discussion

Two themes were identified through the data gathering and analysis. The first was the importance of partnership working, and its direct and indirect benefits for schools and clubs. Despite the fact that, on the whole, reports of partnership working from both head teachers and community managers were positive, there did appear to be scope for more formalization within the partnerships to help better realize their potential.

The second theme was the pivotal role of the community coaches, who acted as mediators and brokers for the partnership, as well as being the most obvious embodiment of the partnership in action. Judgements about the quality and success of the delivery of the programmes relied significantly on the perceived quality of the coaches working with schools. There seems little doubt that recognition of the importance of quality coaching running in parallel with an acknowledgement of the deficiencies of much PESS that would otherwise have been delivered by non-specialist teachers. The implications of this in terms of coach education and continuing professional development are obvious. However, we would also suggest that these findings highlight the absolute necessity of using programmes like this as vehicles for the professional up-skilling of non-specialist teachers, if they are to result in sustainable improvement and development.

The two themes offer an important insight, given the lack of information on the implementation of PESS for young people and the potential importance of PESS to the development of lifelong participation.

Partnerships, or more specifically effective partnerships, require quality coaches. But to extend this further, it was apparent that coaching practice and professional football clubs were unable to evidence impact and quality to inform head teacher decision-making. To evidence impact and/or quality could impact the development and sustainability of partnerships. Once consideration could be total quality management (TQM), which is an approach whereby all organizational members work towards achieving quality standards.[45] This involves a focus on customer satisfaction, continuous improvement and total involvement. Research and evaluation within TQM is key to continued improvement. It was apparent that there was a significant lack of monitoring and evaluation on the role of the coach and the outcomes of PESS delivery. This is a significant weakness, and threatens to undermine both on-going improvement, and an honest appraisal that differentiates what works from what is perceived to work.[46] This may also hinder the development of more effective practice and in turn a drive towards continual improvement.[47]

Within the current PESS landscape funding often can be short-term in nature, football clubs and schools must endeavour to develop their operations to include research and evaluation to satisfy funders and commissioners.[48] In this regard, it is important to adopt both process and impact evaluations that are planned from the outset.[49] This may involve partnering with an academic institute to provide this expertise.[50] This is also supported by NICE, who endorses the need to develop research and evaluation in understanding intervention for children and young people.[51]

The coach was perceived positively by the schools, commenting on their quality, expertise and ability to support the objectives of PESS. The evidence of the importance of coaching quality is associated with continued professional development, which in past research into community coaches has been pinpointed as an area that requires more strategic and coordinated management.[52] Interestingly, both the schools and football clubs found that their partnership involved professional development for and from both the teachers and community coaches. Despite this, some teachers highlighted that not all community coaches were fully prepared. In a study of a football-based school intervention, delivered by a professional football clubs across 4 schools and 57 primary school children, it was found that despite overwhelming support and approval for the community coaches (and the football club) there were elements of poor practice. Interestingly, this was unnoticed, unrecognized and unmonitored by either the football club or the schools involved. This research also highlighted a greater need for monitoring and evaluation.[53]

This level of expertise of the coaches, identified by the head teachers links to NICE guidance for promoting PA in children and young people through relevant leadership and instruction.[54] NICE offers 15 recommendations all of which offer resonance for schools who play a major contributing role in children and young peoples' lives. Indeed, recommendations highlight the need to develop multi-component school and community programmes, as such the development of partnerships to deliver PESS with football clubs will play a key part in this. As such it appears that local partnerships between professional football clubs and schools can play a contributing role in the pursuit of supporting NICE,[55] especially in the absence of the SSP.[56] Indeed, professional football clubs highlighted that they may have now indirectly picked up some of the roles of responsibilities within the new the PE and Sport Premium era. The coach was highlighted emphatically as a successful component of the partnership. Successful partnerships have been highlighted as efficient, predictable and dependable in a way that resources are shared, how the partnership is managed and how the goals are delivered.[57] This partnership was ultimately needs driven through the provision of coaching.[58]

Conclusion

There is very little known about the implementation and partnerships involved in PESS, especially within the new PE and Sport Premium funding era. This research offers an insight into the delivery and partnerships involved. Amongst the growth in external providers of PESS for schools, it is clear that there are a number of partnerships developed between professional football clubs and schools. There appears to be an opportunity to develop the scope of these partnerships more formally to capitalize on the indirect outcomes, notably mutual continued professional development. Quality coaching is the key factor in the development and perceived effectiveness of the partnerships. As such, the development of continued professional development and quality assurance measures for community coaches would be critical to developing effective practice and partnerships. It was clear that the partnerships would also benefit from the monitoring and evaluation of coaching practice, which is currently absent. There is a need for process and impact evaluation on the PESS outcomes. The lack of monitoring and evaluation is something that must be remedied to enhance the understanding, the effectiveness and impact of the partnerships, in order to improve practice and the subsequent effectiveness of PESS. Given increased investment from strategic stakeholders such as The Premier League, it is vital that professional football clubs work towards enacting these positive changes. Without this, we can only speculate on how PESS can contribute lifelong participation in children and young people.

Acknowledgements

The authors would like to thank all participants from the schools and professional football clubs for their access, time and importantly insight into this research area. To Angus Martin of the Football League Trust for his cooperation with the research process. Thank you to Simone Buchaeser and Rebecca Adams for their engagement with the research process.

Disclosure statement

No potential conflict of interest was reported by the authors.

Notes

1. Philpotts and Grix, 'New Governance and Physical Education and School Sport Policy: A Case Study of School to Club Links'.
2. Siedentop, Hastie, and Van der Mars, *Complete Guide to Sport Education*.
3. National Institute for Health and Care Excellence, 'Promoting Physical Activity for Children and Young People'.
4. Bull and Bauman, 'Physical Inactivity: The "Cinderella" Risk Factor for Noncommunicable Disease Prevention'; Crook et al., 'Does Human Capital Matter? A Meta-analysis of the Relationship between Human Capital and Firm Performance'; and Kohl et al., 'The Pandemic of Physical Inactivity: Global Action for Public Health'.
5. World Health Organization, *Facing the Facts #1: Chronic Diseases and Their Common Risk Factors*; Olshansky et al., 'A Potential Decline in Life Expectancy of the United States in the 21st Century'; Fernandes and Zanesco, 'Early Physical Activity Promotes Lower Prevalence of Chronic Diseases in Adulthood'; and Craigie et al., 'Tracking of Obesity-related Behaviours from Childhood to Adulthood: A Systematic Review'.
6. Kipping, Jago, and Lawlor, 'Obesity in Children. Part 1: Epidemiology, Measurement, Risk Factors, and Screening'.
7. Bailey et al., 'Physical Activity: An Underestimated Investment in Human Capital?'.
8. National Institute for Health and Care Excellence, 'Promoting Physical Activity for Children and Young People'.
9. Ibid.
10. Siedentop, Hastie, and Van der Mars, *Complete Guide to Sport Education*.
11. Kirk and Gorely, 'Challenging Thinking about the Relationship between School Physical Education and Sport Performance'; Philpotts and Grix, 'New Governance and Physical Education and School Sport Policy: A Case Study of School to Club Links'.
12. Department for Education and Skills/Department for Culture Media and Sport, *Learning through PE and Sport: A Guide to the Physical Education, School Sport and Club Link Strategy*.
13. Department for Culture Media and Sport, *Playing to Win: A New Era for Sport*.
14. Phillpots, 'An Analysis of the Policy Process for Physical Education and School Sport: The Rise and Demise of School Sport Partnerships'.
15. London Organising Committee of the Olympic and Paralympic Games, 'Olympic Games Concept and Legacy'; London Organising Committee of the Olympic and Paralympic Games, 'Everyone's Games'.
16. National Audit Office, 'Measuring up: How Good are the Government's Data Systems for Monitoring Performance against Public Service Agreements? Review of the Data Systems for Public Service Agreement 22'.
17. British Olympic Association, *London Olympic Bid; Candidature File*; Department for Culture Media and Sport, *Legacy Action Plans: Before, During and After: Making the Most of the London 2012 Games*.
18. Parnell, Millward, and Spracklen, 'Sport and Austerity in the UK: An Insight into Liverpool 2014'.
19. Philpotts and Grix, 'New Governance and Physical Education and School Sport policy: A Case Study of School to Club Links'.
20. Ibid.
21. Department for Culture Media and Sport, *Creating a Sporting Habit for Life: A New Youth Sport Strategy*.
22. Ibid.
23. The Premier League, 'Premier League Investing to Support PE and Sports in Primary Schools'.
24. Parnell and Richardson, 'Introduction: Football and Inclusivity'.
25. Parnell et al., 'Football in the Community Schemes: Exploring the Effectiveness of an Intervention in Promoting Healthful Behaviour Change'.
26. Watson, 'Football in the Community: "What's the Score?"'; Brown, Crabbe, and Mellor, '*Football and Its Communities: Final Report*'; Parnell et al., 'Football in the Community Schemes: Exploring the Effectiveness of an Intervention in Promoting Healthful Behaviour Change'; Anagnostopoulos and Shilbury, 'Implementing Corporate

Social Responsibility in English Football: Towards Multi-theoretical Integration'; and Parnell and Richardson, 'Introduction: Football and Inclusivity'.

27. Walters and Panton, 'Corporate Social Responsibility and Social Partnerships in Professional Football'.

28. Bingham et al., 'Fit Fans: Perspectives of a Practitioner and Understanding Participant Health Needs within a Health Promotion Programme for Older Men Delivered within an English Premier League Football Club'; Curran et al., 'Ethnographic Engagement from within a Football in the Community Programme at an English Premier League Football Club'; Hunt et al., 'A Gender-sensitized Weight Loss and Healthy Living Programme for Overweight and Obese Men Delivered by Scottish Premier League Football Clubs (FFIT): A Pragmatic Randomised Controlled Trial'; Pringle, McKenna, and Zwolinsky, 'An Even More Beautiful Game'; Pringle, McKenna, and Zwolinsky, 'Health Improvement and Professional Football: Players on the Same Side?'; and Pringle et al., 'Effect of a National Programme of Men's Health Delivered in English Premier League Football Clubs'.

29. Rutherford et al., '"Motivate": The Effect of a Football in the Community Delivered Weight Loss Programme on over 35-year Old Men and Women's Cardiovascular Risk Factors'.

30. Curran et al., 'Ethnographic Engagement from within a Football in the Community Programme at an English Premier League Football Club'.

31. Pringle et al., 'Effect of a Health Improvement Programme for Older Adults Delivered in/by Burton Albion FC'; Parnell et al., 'Reaching Older People with Physical Activity Delivered in Football Clubs: The Reach, Adoption and Implementation Characteristics of the Extra Time Programme'.

32. Kiernan and Porter, 'Little United and the Big Society: Negotiating the Gaps between Football, Community and the Politics of Inclusion'; Paramio Salcines, Grady, and Downs, 'Growing the Football Game: The Increasing Economic and Social Relevance of Older Fans and Those with Disabilities in the European Football Industry'.

33. Parnell et al., 'Understanding Football as a Vehicle for Enhancing Social Inclusion: Using an Intervention Mapping Framework'.

34. The Premier League, 'Premier League Investing to Support PE and Sports in Primary Schools'.

35. Babiak and Wolfe, 'More Than Just a Game? Corporate Social Responsibility and Super Bowl XL', Anagnostopoulos and Shilbury, 'Implementing Corporate Social Responsibility in English Football: Towards Multi-theoretical Integration'; and Parnell and Richardson, 'Introduction: Football and Inclusivity'.

36. National Institute for Health and Care Excellence, 'Promoting Physical Activity for Children and Young People'.

37. Parnell et al., 'Football in the Community Schemes: Exploring the Effectiveness of an Intervention in Promoting Healthful Behaviour Change'; Parnell et al., 'Implementing "Monitoring and Evaluation" Techniques within a Premier League Football in the Community Scheme'.

38. Babiak, 'Determinants of Interorganizational Relationships: The Case of a Canadian Nonprofit Sport Organization'; O'Reilly and Brunette, 'Public–Private Partnerships in Physical Activity and Sport'.

39. The Football League Trust.

40. Philpotts and Grix, 'New Governance and Physical Education and School Sport Policy: A Case Study of School to Club Links'; Bailey et al., 'Physical Activity: An Underestimated Investment in Human Capital?'; Kirk and Gorely, 'Challenging Thinking about the Relationship between School Physical Education and Sport Performance'; and Parnell et al., 'Football in the Community Schemes: Exploring the Effectiveness of an Intervention in Promoting Healthful Behaviour Change'.

41. Walters and Panton, 'Corporate Social Responsibility and Social Partnerships in Professional Football'; Babiak, 'Determinants of Interorganizational Relationships: The Case of a Canadian Nonprofit Sport Organization'; and O'Reilly and Brunette, 'Public–Private Partnerships in Physical Activity and Sport'.

42. National Institute for Health and Care Excellence, 'Promoting Physical Activity for Children and Young People'.

43. Strauss and Corbin, *Basics of Qualitative Research: Techniques and Procedures for Developing Grounded Theory.*
44. Parnell et al., 'Football in the Community Schemes: Exploring the Effectiveness of an Intervention in Promoting Healthful Behaviour Change'.
45. De Knop, Hoecke, and Bosscher, 'Quality Management in Sports Clubs'.
46. Parnell et al., 'Implementing "Monitoring and Evaluation" Techniques within a Premier League Football in the Community Scheme'; Pringle et al., 'Assessing the Impact of Football-based Health Improvement Programmes: Stay Onside, Avoid Own Goals and Bag the Evaluation'.
47. Babiak and Thibault, 'Challenges in Multiple Cross-sector Partnerships'; De Knop, Hoecke, and Bosscher, 'Quality Management in Sports Clubs'.
48. Babiak and Thibault, 'Challenges in Multiple Cross-sector Partnerships'; Pringle, McKenna, and Zwolinsky, 'Health Improvement and Professional Football: Players on the Same Side?'.
49. Pringle et al., 'Assessing the Impact of Football-based Health Improvement Programmes: Stay Onside, Avoid Own Goals and Bag the Evaluation'.
50. Parnell et al., 'Understanding Football as a Vehicle for Enhancing Social Inclusion: Using an Intervention Mapping Framework'.
51. National Institute for Health and Care Excellence, 'Promoting Physical Activity for Children and Young People'.
52. Parnell et al., 'Football in the Community Schemes: Exploring the Effectiveness of an Intervention in Promoting Healthful Behaviour Change'.
53. Ibid.
54. National Institute for Health and Care Excellence, 'Promoting Physical Activity for Children and Young People'.
55. Ibid.
56. Phillpots, 'An Analysis of the Policy Process for Physical Education and School Sport: The Rise and Demise of School Sport Partnerships'.
57. Babiak, 'Determinants of Interorganizational Relationships: The Case of a Canadian Nonprofit Sport Organization'.
58. O'Reilly and Brunette, 'Public–Private Partnerships in Physical Activity and Sport'.

References

Anagnostopoulos, C., and D. Shilbury. 'Implementing Corporate Social Responsibility in English Football: Towards Multi-theoretical Integration'. *Sport, Business and Management: An International Journal* 3, no. 4 (2013): 268–84.

Babiak, K. 'Determinants of Interorganizational Relationships: The Case of a Canadian Nonprofit Sport Organization'. *Journal of Sport Management* 21, no. 3 (2007): 338–76.

Babiak, K., and L. Thibault. 'Challenges in Multiple Cross-sector Partnerships'. *Nonprofit and Voluntary Sector Quarterly* 38, no. 1 (2009): 117–43.

Babiak, K., and R. Wolfe. 'More than Just a Game? Corporate Social Responsibility and Super Bowl XL'. *Sport Marketing Quarterly* 15, no. 4 (2006): 214–24.

Bailey, R., C. Hillman., S. Arent, and A. Petitpas. 'Physical Activity: An Underestimated Investment in Human Capital?' *Journal of Physical Activity and Health* 10 (2013): 289–308.

Bingham, D.D., D. Parnell, K. Curran, R. Jones, and D. Richardson. 'Fit Fans: Perspectives of a Practitioner and Understanding Participant Health Needs within a Health Promotion Programme for Older Men Delivered within an English Premier League Football Club'. *Soccer & Society* 15, no. 6 (2014): 883–901.

British Olympic Association. *London Olympic Bid; Candidature File*. London: BOA, 2004.

Brown, A., T. Crabbe, and G. Mellor. *Football and Its Communities: Final Report*. London: Football Foundation and Manchester Metropolitan University, 2006.

Bull, F.C., and A.E. Bauman. 'Physical Inactivity: The "Cinderella" Risk Factor for Non-communicable Disease Prevention'. *Journal of Health Communication: International Perspectives* 16, suppl 2 (2011): 13–26.

Craigie, A., A. Lake, S. Kelly, A. Adamson, and J. Mathers. 'Tracking of Obesity-related Behaviours from Childhood to Adulthood: A Systematic Review'. *Maturitas* 70, no. 3 (2011): 266–84.

Crook, T.R., S.Y. Todd, J.G. Combs, D.J. Woehr, and D.J. Ketchen. 'Does Human Capital Matter? A Meta-analysis of the Relationship between Human Capital and Firm Performance'. *Journal of Applied Psychology* 96, no. 3 (2011): 443–56.

Curran, K., D. Bingham, D. Richardson, and D. Parnell. 'Ethnographic Engagement from within a Football in the Community Programme at an English Premier League Football Club'. *Soccer & Society* 15 (2014): 934–50.

De Knop, P., J.V. Hoecke, and V.D. Bosscher. 'Quality Management in Sports Clubs'. *Sport Management Review* 7 (2004): 55–77.

Department for Culture Media and Sport. *Legacy Action Plans: Before, during and after: Making the Most of the London 2012 Games*. London: DCMS, 2008.

Department for Culture Media and Sport. *Playing to Win: A New Era for Sport*. London: DCMS, 2008.

Department for Culture Media and Sport. *Creating a Sporting Habit for Life: A New Youth Sport Strategy*. London: DCMS, 2012.

Department for Education and Skills/Department for Culture Media and Sport. *Learning through PE and Sport: A Guide to the Physical Education, School Sport and Club Link Strategy*. London: Department for Education and Skills, 2003.

Fernandes, R., and A. Zanesco. 'Early Physical Activity Promotes Lower Prevalence of Chronic Diseases in Adulthood'. *Hypertension Research* 33 (2010): 926–31.

The Football League Trust. 2015. http://www.football-league.co.uk/global/aboutfltrust.aspx (accessed January 10, 2015).

Hunt, K., S. Wyke, C. Gray, A. Anderson, A. Brady, C. Bunn, P.T. Donnon et al. 'A Gender-sensitised Weight Loss and Healthy Living Programme for Overweight and Obese Men Delivered by Scottish Premier League Football Clubs (FFIT): A Pragmatic Randomised Controlled Trial'. *The Lancet* 383 (2014): 1211–21.

Kiernan. A and P. Porter. 'Little United and the Big Society: Negotiating the Gaps between Football, Community and the Politics of Inclusion'. *Soccer & Society* 15, no. 6 (2014): 847–63.

Kipping, R., R. Jago, and D. Lawlor. 'Obesity in Children. Part 1: Epidemiology, Measurement, Risk Factors, and Screening'. *BMJ* 337 (2008): 922–7.

Kirk, D., and T. Gorely. 'Challenging Thinking about the Relationship between School Physical Education and Sport Performance'. *European Physical Education Review* 6, no. 2 (2000): 119–34.

Kohl, H.W., C.L. Craig, E.W. Lambert, S. Inoue, J.R. Alkandari, G. Leetongin, and S. Kahlmeier. 'The Pandemic of Physical Inactivity: Global Action for Public Health'. *Lancet* 330 (2012): 294–305.

London Organising Committee of the Olympic and Paralympic Games. 'Everyone's Games'. 2007. http://www.london2012.com/documents/locog-publications/everyones-games.pdf (accessed February 20, 2015).

London Organising Committee of the Olympic and Paralympic Games. 'Olympic Games Concept and Legacy'. 2007. http://www.london2012.com/publications/theme-1-olympic-games-concept-and-legacy.ph (accessed February 20, 2015).

National Audit Office. 'Measuring up: How Good are the Government's Data Systems for Monitoring Performance against Public Service Agreements?' *Review of the Data Systems for Public Service Agreement* 22 (2010). http://www.nao.org.uk/publications/1011/review_data_systems_for_psa_22.aspx (accessed February 20, 2015).

National Institute for Health and Care Excellence. 'Promoting Physical Activity for Children and Young People'. 2009. https://www.nice.org.uk/guidance/ph17 (accessed January 10, 2015).

Olshansky, S.J., D.J. Passaro, R.C. Hershow, J. Layden, B.A. Carnes, J. Brody, L. Hayflick, R.N. Butler, D.B. Allison, and D.S. Ludwig. 'A Potential Decline in Life Expectancy of the United States in the 21st Century'. *The New England Journal of Medicine* 352, no. 11 (2005): 1138–45.

O'Reilly, N., and M.K. Brunette. 'Public–Private Partnerships in Physical Activity and Sport'. *Human Kinetics*. (2014). http://www.humankinetics.com/products/all-products/public-private-partnerships-in-physical-activity-and-sport

Paramio Salcines, J.L., J. Grady, and P. Downs. 'Growing the Football Game: The Increasing Economic and Social Relevance of Older Fans and Those with Disabilities in the European Football Industry'. *Soccer & Society* 15, no. 6 (2014): 864–82.

Parnell, D., P. Millward, and K. Spracklen. 'Sport and Austerity in the UK: An Insight into Liverpool 2014'. *Journal of Policy Research in Tourism, Leisure and Events* 7, no. 2 (2014): 200–3. doi: 10.1080/19407963.2014.968309.

Parnell, D., A. Pringle, P. Widdop, and S. Zwolinsky. 'Understanding Football as a Vehicle for Enhancing Social Inclusion: Using an Intervention Mapping Framework'. *Social Inclusion* 3, no. 3 (2015): 158–66.

Parnell, D., A. Pringle, S. Zwolinsky, J. McKenna, Z. Rutherford, D. Richardson, L. Trotter, M. Rigby, and M.J. Hargreaves. 'Reaching Older People with Physical Activity Delivered in Football Clubs: The Reach, Adoption and Implementation Characteristics of the Extra Time Programme'. *BMC Public Health* 15 (2015). doi: 10.1186/s12889-015-1560-5. http://www.biomedcentral.com/1471-2458/15/220

Parnell, D., and D. Richardson. 'Introduction: Football and Inclusivity'. *Soccer & Society* 15, no. 6 (2014): 823–7.

Parnell, D., G. Stratton, B. Drust, and D. Richardson. 'Football in the Community Schemes: Exploring the Effectiveness of an Intervention in Promoting Healthful Behaviour Change'. *Soccer & Society* 14 (2013): 35–51.

Parnell, D., G. Stratton, B. Drust, and D. Richardson. 'Implementing "Monitoring and Evaluation" Techniques within a Premier League Football in the Community Scheme'. In *Routledge Handbook of Sport and Social Responsibility*, ed. Juan Luis Paramio Salcines, Kathy Babiak, and Geoff Walters, 328–43. London: Routledge, 2013.

Phillpots, L. 'An Analysis of the Policy Process for Physical Education and School Sport: The Rise and Demise of School Sport Partnerships'. *International Journal of Sport Policy and Politics* 5, no. 2 (2013): 193–211.

Philpotts, L., and J. Grix. 'New Governance and Physical Education and School Sport Policy: A Case Study of School to Club Links'. *Physical Education and Sport Pedagogy* 19, no. 1 (2014): 76–96.

Pringle, A., J. McKenna, and S. Zwolinsky. 'An Even More Beautiful Game'. *Public Health* 127 (2013): 1143–4.

Pringle, A., J. McKenna, and S. Zwolinsky. 'Health Improvement and Professional Football: Players on the Same Side?' *Journal of Policy Research in Tourism Leisure and Events* 5 (2013): 207–12.

Pringle, A., D. Parnell, S. Zwolinsky, J. Hargreaves, and J. McKenna. 'Effect of a Health Improvement Programme for Older Adults Delivered in/by Burton Albion FC'. *Soccer & Society* 15, no. 6 (2014): 902–18.

Pringle, A., S. Zwolinsky, J. Hargreaves, L. Lozano, and J. McKenna. 'Assessing the Impact of Football-based Health Improvement Programmes: Stay Onside, Avoid Own Goals and Bag the Evaluation'. *Soccer & Society* 15, no. 2 (2014): 970–87.

Pringle, A., S. Zwolinsky, J. McKenna, A. Daly-Smith, S. Robertson, and A. White. 'Effect of a National Programme of Men's Health Delivered in English Premier League Football Clubs'. *Public Health* 127 (2013): 18–26.

Rutherford, Z., B. Gough, S. Seymour-Smith, C. Matthews, J. WIlcox, D. Parnell. '"Motivate": The Effect of a Football in the Community Delivered Weight Loss Programme on over 35-year Old Men and Women's Cardiovascular Risk Factors'. *Soccer & Society* 16 (2014): 951–69.

Siedentop, D., P. Hastie, and H. Van der Mars, eds. *Complete Guide to Sport Education*. Champaign, IL: Human Kinetics, 2004.

Strauss, A., and J. Corbin. *Basics of Qualitative Research: Techniques and Procedures for Developing Grounded Theory*. 2nd ed. Thousand Oaks, CA: Sage, 1998.

The Premier League. 'Premier League Investing to Support PE and Sports in Primary Schools'. 2014. http://www.premierleague.com/en-gb/communities/2014-15/premier-league-major-investment-in-primary-school-pe-and-sport.html (accessed February 15, 2015).

Walters, G., and M. Panton. 'Corporate Social Responsibility and Social Partnerships in Professional Football'. *Soccer & Society* 15, no. 6 (2014): 828–46.

Watson, N. 'Football in the Community: "What's the Score?"'. *Soccer & Society* 1, no. 1 (2000): 114–25.

World Health Organization. *Facing the Facts #1: Chronic Diseases and Their Common Risk Factors*, Geneva: World Health Organisation. 2005.

Can 'English Premier League' funding for PE and school sport achieve its aims?

Stephen Zwolinsky, Jim McKenna, Daniel Parnell and Andy Pringle

Centre for Active Lifestyles, Institute of Sport, Physical Activity and Leisure, Leeds Beckett University, Leeds, UK

There are a number of assertions being made for a £10 m investment by the English Premier League for primary school sport. For example, it is claimed that Physical Education plus school sport can improve cognitive functioning, concentration, behaviour, educational attainment and overall physical health. However, far from being sufficient in helping to achieve these benefits and sustain long-term activity participation, for some children, Physical Education and competitive sport may actually be counterproductive. In some instances, it may switch them off from activity altogether. Therefore, we need to understand more about which elements of this scheme work, who they work for and which circumstances they work in. Fundamentally, this will only be achieved through hard evidence and robust evaluation.

In 2014, the English Premier League (EPL) announced £10 m funding for a three-year programme (2104–2017) of primary school sport across the country.[1] This engendered a mixed response; the EPL was enthusiastic about the timing and size of this £10 m investment, while some members of the press labelled it as a PR stunt, comparing the funding to the vast expenditure of EPL clubs in player transfer fees.[2] Critics didn't reserve reproach for the EPL, detractors also questioned the propriety of any collection of private companies filling the void left by the government's underfunding of Physical Education (PE) and school sport.[3] To this end, the UK Sport approach to funding was also drawn in; they were accused of 'Olympic medal hunting'. They were also suspected of ignoring the majority of the population, who are both under-active and incapable of achieving any benchmarks for sporting eliteness.[4] With these thoughts in mind, it is worth taking a closer look at the assertions being made for the EPL's school sports scheme.

In business, market forces often drive large investments supported by easy and slick lines of argument using imprecise and exaggerated claims. In this instance, the EPL might reasonably claim that it is giving the schools and school children what they want and how they want it.[5] However, the rhetoric around the EPL investment is hyped and metaphorically, it is important that advocates have their feet held to the fire for the big claims they make. One problem of the imprecision underpinning these big claims is that they – quite wrongly – conflate PE with school sport to claim that 'they' (i.e. PE plus school sports) improve participants' cognitive functioning, concentration, behaviour, overall physical health and educational attainment.[6] Isn't it more reasonable to expect that the different experiences that PE and school sport might represent will bring about distinctive outcomes? Equally, it would be more compelling if the evidence showed that it was the programme – and not some tangential, coincidental change – that produced any increase in physical activity. Without empirical evidence, assumptions that primary school PE – which is limited to life before age 12 – or involvement in sport – which is little more than a distant memory for most over 40 years of age[7] – will help to tackle the onset of major lifestyle diseases appear hyperbolic.

Moreover, the evidence that underpins many of the claims made for this new scheme has only been previously linked to regular and sustained involvement in physical activity.[8] Ironically, on their own, PE lessons rarely produce the levels of physical activity required to generate these benefits.[9] Indeed, there is ample short-term evidence to show that the structure and content of PE is often unsuccessful in helping children accumulate enough of the moderate to vigorous intensity physical activity (MVPA) that enhances health. At present, children and young people (5–18 years) are recommended to engage in 60 min of MVPA each day.[10] Further, there are limitations regarding the effectiveness of coaches working in schools, for delivering on the health agenda.[11] Indeed, even when academics have strictly controlled two hours of 'quality' MVPA, the evidence is inconclusive that any of the 'big' claims made for the EPL investment are achievable.[12] In essence, neither PE nor school sport is sufficiently structured to develop lifelong activity participation.

To compound this, the experiences of physical activity that stem from organised school sport and PE seem to have been central to switching off many of our long-term inactive people from any form of exercise.[13] Central to these aversive experiences are those relating to competition and to handling high levels of unaccustomed exertion.[14] This is compounded when activities entail social judgements of competence and social standing. For many inactive individuals, this alone is a powerful reason not to engage. Therefore, offering more sport to individuals who don't like sport is rarely, if ever, the answer to their inactivity. Worse, it may be helping to drive the modern day epidemic of inactivity. In this understanding, it is difficult to envisage how the promotion of competitive sport will meet the needs of even a sizeable minority of our under-active individuals.

Nevertheless, emerging findings from this school sports programme have suggested that it has already 'delivered more than 66,000 PE lessons and sport sessions in 1279 schools to over 103,000 pupils'.[15] While this seems impressive, two important questions remain: Which of the specific big claims is this delivering and what proportion of young people feel and have actually accrued these benefits from their involvement? To answer these questions, it would have required that funders and stakeholders invest in quality evaluation specifically designed to establish impact. Furthermore, these investigations should not only evaluate outcomes, but also the process by which the impact occurs.[16] It is important to address the 'active ingredients' that make this happen to find out which elements work and which don't. Evaluators need to detail how programmes develop and progress year-on-year, and then show the hard evidence that confirms what the investment has achieved. Only when that's clear can we understand these big claims more accurately.

Additionally, evaluation should be integral to intervention design and made part of intervention mapping;[17] too often, evaluation is included as an afterthought. Where interventions lack a robust evaluation, they risk failing to identify the overall panoply of outcomes, including those that are hard to anticipate and/or hazardous to overlook. This ill-advised practice means that stakeholders can end up making approximations and assumptions about 'outcomes' that are much cruder and far more unrefined than we might initially realise. School sport is replete with examples where stakeholders, using half-baked evidence from previous interventions, invest in what looks to be a powerful programme. Too often, that ends with an awkward, whispered acknowledgement that the financial investment has been squandered.

Yet, there is much good in promoting physical activity, exercise and health through football. As the national game, and notwithstanding the massive spectatorship that it generates, it also supports extensive – if declining – levels of exercise in community settings.[18] Ultimately, most people aspire to live well – whether or not this involves leading a healthy lifestyle – and to have the functional capacity to go about their daily lives. These are not incompatible goals and in many circumstances, these goals have the potential to be mediated through an active lifestyle fostered while at school. Schemes like that, established by the EPL investment, are desirable to children because they are 'designer' or 'branded', which implies that they represent an innovative approach. However, in these circumstances, the level of engagement they create may only last as long as the fashion cycle. Yet, to support inactive individuals in becoming more active, it is helpful to think more of a 'perpetual purchase', rather than encouraging the pursuit of the latest trend. To do this, we need to establish effectiveness and determine the possible effects of taking action or not. In the long run, there will always be a little bit of uncertainty because there are some processes that we don't fully understand, but we measure scientific progress by our ability to reduce the uncertainty and by that yardstick, there is plenty of room for improvement.

Disclosure statement

No potential conflict of interest was reported by the authors.

Notes

1. The Premier League, 'Premier League Investing to Support PE and Sports in Primary Schools'.
2. Moore, 'Private Clubs should not be Expected to Plug the Gaps in Basic State Provision'.
3. Phillpots and Grix, 'New Governance and Physical Education and School Sport Policy: A Case Study of School to Club Links'.
4. Moore, 'Private Clubs should not be Expected to Plug the Gaps in Basic State Provision'.
5. Ibid.
6. The Premier League, 'Premier League Investing to Support PE and Sports in Primary Schools'.
7. Sport England, 'Active People Survey'.
8. Department of Health, *Start Active Stay Active*.
9. Fairclough and Stratton, 'A Review of Physical Activity Levels during Elementary School Education'.
10. Department of Health, *Start Active Stay Active*.
11. Parnell et al., 'Football in the Community Schemes: Exploring the Effectiveness of an Intervention in Promoting Healthful Behaviour Change'.
12. van Sluijs, McMinn, and Griffin, 'Effectiveness of Interventions to Promote Physical Activity in Children and Adolescents: Systematic Review of Controlled Trials'; and Lonsdale et al., 'A Systematic Review and Meta-analysis of Interventions Designed to

Increase Moderate-to-vigorous Physical Activity in School Physical Education Lessons'.
13. Robson and McKenna, *Sports and Health*.
14. Ibid.
15. The Premier League, 'Premier League Investing to Support PE and Sports in Primary Schools'.
16. Pringle et al., 'Health Improvement for Men and Hard-to-engage-men Delivered in English Premier League Football Clubs'.
17. Ransdell et al., *Developing Effective Physical Activity Programmes*.
18. Zwolinsky et al., 'Optimizing Lifestyles for Men Regarded as "hard-to-reach" through Top-flight Football/soccer Clubs'.

References

Department of Health. *Start Active, Stay Active: A Report on Physical Activity for Health from the Four Home Countries*. Chief Medical Officers. London: Department of Health, 2011.

Fairclough, S., and G. Stratton. 'A Review of Physical Activity Levels during Elementary School Education'. *Journal of Teaching and Physical Education* 25, no. 2 (2006): 239–57.

Lonsdale, C., R. Rosenkranz, L. Peralta, A. Bennie, P. Fahey, and D. Lubans. 'A Systematic Review and Meta-Analysis of Interventions Designed to Increase Moderate-to-Vigorous Physical Activity in School Physical Education Lessons'. *Preventive Medicine* 56, no. 2 (2013): 152–61.

Moore, G. 'Private Clubs should not be Expected to Plug the Gaps in Basic State Provision'. *The Independent*, 2014. http://www.independent.co.uk/sport/football/premier-league/private-clubs-should-not-be-expected-to-plug-the-gaps-in-basic-state-provision-9664929.html (accessed September 9, 2014).

Parnell, D., G. Stratton, B. Drust, and D. Richardson. 'Football in the Community Schemes: Exploring the Effectiveness of an Intervention in Promoting Healthful Behaviour Change'. *Soccer & Society* 14 (2013): 35–51.

Phillpots, L., and J. Grix. 'New Governance and Physical Education and School Sport Policy: A Case Study of School to Club Links'. *Physical Education and Sport Pedagogy* 19, no. 1 (2014): 76–96.

The Premier League. 'Premier League Investing to Support PE and Sports in Primary Schools'. 2014. http://www.premierleague.com/en-gb/communities/2014-15/premier-league-major-investment-in-primary-school-pe-and-sport.html (accessed February 15, 2015).

Pringle, A., S. Zwolinsky, J. McKenna, S. Robertson, A. Daly-Smith, and A. White. 'Health Improvement for Men and Hard-to-engage-men Delivered in English Premier League Football Clubs'. *Health Education Research* 29, no. 3 (2014): 503–20.

Ransdell, L., M. Dinger, J. Huberty, and K. Miller. *Developing Effective Physical Activity Programmes*. Champaign, IL: Human Kinetics, 2009.

Robson, S., and J. McKenna. 'Sports and Health'. In *Sports Development: Policy, Process and Practice*, ed. K Hylton, 3rd ed., 173–94. London: Routledge, 2013.

van Sluijs, E., A. McMinn, and S. Griffin. 'Effectiveness of Interventions to Promote Physical Activity in Children and Adolescents: Systematic Review of Controlled Trials'. *British Journal of Sports Medicine* 42, no. 8 (2008): 653–7.

Sport England. 'Active People Survey 7–12 months Rolling Results: April 2012–April 2013'. http://www.sportengland.org/research/who-plays-sport/national-picture/ (accessed August 3, 2014).

Zwolinsky, S., J. McKenna, A. Pringle, A. Daly-Smith, S. Robertson, and A. White. 'Optimizing Lifestyles for Men Regarded as 'hard-to-reach' through Top-Flight Football/Soccer Clubs'. *Health Education Research* 28, no. 3 (2013): 405–13.

The influence of club football on children's daily physical activity

Glen Nielsen[a,c], Anna Bugge[b,c] and Lars Bo Andersen[b,c]

[a]Center for Team Sports and Health, Department of Nutrition, Exercise and Sports Sciences, University of Copenhagen, Copenhagen, Denmark; [b]Center for Research in Childhood Health, University of Southern Denmark, Odense, Denmark; [c]Department of Sports Medicine, Norwegian School of Sport Sciences, Oslo, Norway

Studies on the effects of organized club sports on children's total amount of physical activity (PA) show varying results. This may be partly due to different sports having different activity levels, but also different possibilities for being played outside club settings. This study investigates how playing football as a club sport is associated to the total amount of daily PA among children and how increased school recess activity impacts on this. Using accelerometers, the average daily amount of children's PA as well the activity levels in specific contexts, such as during club-sports and school recess, was measured on a sample of 518 Danish children aged 9–10. The study found that children playing club football had higher total daily amounts of PA than both children taking part in other club-sports and children not taking part in club-sports at all. About half of the difference in total PA could be explained by higher activity levels during school recess. The association between club football and total PA, and the mediating effect of school recess PA, can be interpreted as the result of two main factors: the high activity levels during club football, and that Danish school grounds have football facilities which allow able and interested children to play football for many hours each week during school recess. On a more general level, the results indicate that the influence leisure-time club sport participation has on PA may differ due to how well the sport can be transferred to and played in other daily contexts for children's self-organized PA, such as school recess.

Introduction

Physical activity (PA) in children has been shown to decrease the level of cardio-vascular disease risk factors and increase bone density.[1] This has made children's overall PA a fundamental part of health promotion policies in many countries.[2] One strategy that is often used in Denmark and other Scandinavian countries is to try to increase the number of children participating in leisure-time club sport.[3] However, studies on the effects of organized club sports on children's total amount of PA show varying results.[4] One study found that participating in club-organized sports did not strongly influence 6–10 year old children's total amount of daily PA, but that activity levels during school recess and other contexts for self-organized play did as children spend many more hours each week in such contexts than they do participating in club sports.[5] It is likely that different sports have different effects and influences on the total amount PA. The influence of club sports on children's total amount of PA may vary due to the differing PA levels involved in different types of sports, but perhaps also due to differences in how well the sport can be transferred to other contexts important for children's self-organized physically active play, such as school recess.

Surveys show that football is a very common leisure-time sport among Danish children, especially for boys.[6,7] Football has been shown to produce high activity levels especially when played in small teams.[8] Studies have also shown that football is a common activity in school recess among boys, and that this activity and its facilities occupy large proportions of Danish school grounds during recess, creating good opportunities for large amounts of daily PA for those children (most often boys) who are able and interested to play.[9] This study tests the hypothesis that football will have a stronger influence on children's daily amount of PA than other types of leisure-time club sports, due partly to the high activity levels when playing football in the club, but especially to increased school recess activity for those children playing the sport. This is done by firstly testing the association between leisure-time club football participation and total amount of daily PA in a large sample of third-grade children, and secondly testing the mediating effect of school break activity levels on this association.

Methods

Participants

Two Danish suburban municipalities – Taarnby and Ballerup – were invited and agreed to participate in a large multidisciplinary study of children's PA called COS-CIS. All 18 schools in these two municipalities agreed to participate. The 1024 children attending third grade in the 18 schools were invited to participate in the study. Seven hundred and four consented to take part. From these 704 participants, questionnaire data combined with sufficient measures of PA[10] were obtained from 518 children when the children were in third grade (9–10 years old). This sample is broadly representative of the general Danish population in terms of social parameters such as the distribution of rental and self-owned accommodation, socio-economic position and the proportion from ethnic minorities.[11]

Measurements of PA

The children's habitual PA was measured using the uniaxial MTI 7164 accelerometers (Actigraph, Fort Walton Beach, Florida, USA). The MTI 7164 accelerometers have been well validated in children against gold standard measures of PA[12] and have been shown to compare favourably with other similar objective measuring instruments.[13] The monitors record body movement as a combined function of the frequency and intensity of the movement allowing detection of normal human motion and rejecting high-frequency vibrations encountered in activities such as car or bus transport. In order to best reflect the distribution of school days and school-free days (weekends and holidays) in school children's lives, both school days and weekend days were included in the measuring period. The four days of recording included 1–2 weekend-days (mean = 1.68). Due to variation in sleeping patterns in children, accelerometer data were analysed for each child from 7 am to 11 pm. To further ensure that the accelerometer measures of daily PA were not corrupted by including data from periods when the accelerometers were not being worn, a program was used to automatically delete missing data (defined as continuous sequences of zeros longer than 10 min which could only be caused by the accelerometer not being worn). This technique has been recommended as an important part of ensuring the reliability of accelerometer data.[14] To reduce the bias from some children not wearing their monitors for the total measuring period, each child's daily minutes of PA were calculated by multiplying the defined daily measuring period for all children (960 min) with the percentage time for which each child was active during their individual total measuring period. To minimize any bias from the novelty of wearing an activity monitor, the MTI monitors were worn by the children for one day before recording. Data were included in the final data-set only if the monitor had recorded more than eight hours of valid recordings a day for at least three days (4 days $n = 379$, 3 days $n = 139$).[15]

Determining the contexts of the activity measurements and identifying club sports participation

The children's class timetables were collected together with self-reported leisure-time activities in order to identify the contexts for the above-described activity measures. The children's class timetables for the days of measuring were used to classify PA measures as activity during school recess, during school in general and during time outside school. A standardized activity self-report questionnaire jointly filled in by parents and children every day during measurement was used to gain information about the time periods for the children's daily leisure-time activities including the exact time they participated in club-organized sport and what kind of sport they participated in during that time. Children who reported having done sports in institutional settings such as sports clubs, dance or riding schools were categorized as participating in club-organized sports and exercise. Children who reported having played football in a club were categorized as playing club football.

Data transformation to PA variables

To obtain information on the activity levels of the children in more specific daily contexts, data were analysed for Total Time (7 am to 11 pm on all the measured days), and for School Time (defined by the schedule of the class, typically weekdays from 8 am to 2 pm). These time periods were then subdivided into more specific contexts for PA such as school recess and leisure-time club sports using the time table of each child's school class and self-reported activities from questionnaire diaries filled out during the days of accelerometer measurements. Time spent in activity of at least moderate intensity (4–6 METS or 2500–5000 counts per minute reflecting medium exertion in an upright position e.g. walking approximately 5.2 km/h) and vigorous intensity (>6 METS or >5000 counts per minute reflecting a high level of exertion in an upright position e.g. running faster than 6.4 km/h) were calculated. The percentage time spent at these activity levels was calculated by dividing the minutes of each measure by the total minutes of recording. The selection of the counts/min cut-off points identifying moderate and vigorous PA was based on a compromise of the recommendations of five different validation studies of accelerometer measures of PA in children.[16]

Defining and categorizing children as being physically active was based on current health-related PA recommendations[17] of one hour a day of activity of at least a moderate level recommended by many health organizations and authorities (including the Danish National Board of Health).

Statistical analysis

All data were analysed using the statistical software program SPSS 22.0. Differences between children participating in club-organized football, children participating in other club-organized sports and children not participating in organized sports measured in continuous variables such as the amount of PA in total in different contexts were tested using ANOVA. Chi-squared tests were used to test differences between groups in categorical data. The analyses of mediators and moderators of differences in PA between those children participating in club football and those who did not were conducted using general linear models or logistic regression, depending on the nature of the dependent PA variables. The 95% confidence intervals for the associations are reported. p-Values less than 0.05 were considered statistically significant and only associations at this minimum level of statistical significance are reported.

Results

Table 1 describes the study sample in terms of number of participants, gender, age, total daily amount of PA, participation in club football and other leisure-time club-organized sports during the period the activity was measured. It shows that 30% of children in the study participated in some type of organized leisure-time club-sports other than football during the period their activity levels were measured. Fourteen per cent of the boys had participated in club football but only 2% of the girls ($p < 0.001$). Boys had a 10% higher daily amount of PA ($p < 0.001$) than girls.

Daily PA among children participating in club football, participating in other club-sports and children not participating in any club-sports

Table 2 outlines the activity levels in different contexts of children who participated in club football, children who participated in other club-sports and children who did not participate in any club-sports during the days their activity levels were measured. ANOVA showed that these categories of club-sports participation were associated with all the measures of total daily amounts of PA and all the measures of PA during school time.

Table 1. Characteristics of the study population.

	Boys	Girls
N	268	249
Mean age (SD)	9.57 (0.37)	9.46 (0.37)
Participated in club sports	29.48%	30.52%
Played club football***	13.81%	2.01%
Participated in other club sports than football***	15.67%	28.51%
Mean daily minutes of MVPA (SD)***	87.19 (28.49)	75.38 (26.81)

***Gender difference significant at $p < 0.001$.

Table 2. Daily amounts of PA among children: who played club football, participated in other club sports and undertook no leisure-time club sports.

	Played club football	Participated in other club sports	No club sports participation
Total			
Activity (min/day)[aa]	101.46 (26.63)[bbb]	82.89 (29.23)	78.75 (27.27)
Moderate activity (min/day)[aa]	70.20 (17.87)[bbb]	58.33 (16.67)	57.19 (17.61)
Vigorous activity (min/day)[aa]	31.26 (12.03)[bb]	24.55 (15.47)[c]	21.56 (11.83)
Active >1 h daily[aa]	97.6%[bb]	81.4%	72.9%
Vigorously active >1.5 h per week[aa]	92.9%	85.0%[c]	75.7%
School time			
Activity (min/day)[aaa]	43.11 (17.31)[bbb]	31.51 (17.03)	30.56 (14.71)
Moderate activity (min/day)[aaa]	27.62 (10.58)[bbb]	20.69 (8.79)	20.43 (8.85)
Vigorous activity (min/day)[aaa]	15.49 (8.87)[bb]	10.82 (9.42)	10.13 (7.12)

Note: Data are presented as mean (SD) except from % being active >1 h/day and % vigorously active >1.5 h/week.
[aa]Difference between the three groups significant at $p < 0.01$.
[aaa]Difference between the three groups significant at $p < 0.001$.
[bb]Difference between children who played football and children doing other sports significant at $p < 0.01$.
[bbb]Difference between children who played football and children doing other sports significant at $p < 0.001$.
[c]Difference between children who participated in club sports other than football and children who didn't participate in any club sport significant at $p < 0.05$.

Children who had participated in club football had a 22% higher total daily amount of PA ($p < 0.001$) and a 27% higher daily amount of vigorous activity ($p = 0.003$) than children who had participated in other club-sports. Only 2% of children playing club football did not reach the recommended 1 h of daily activity; this is significantly less than the 19% of children doing other sports and the 27% of the children not doing any sports. When adjusting for gender, children playing club football had 10.89 higher odds of being physically active more than an hour daily (95% CI: 1.47–80.69, $p = 0.019$).

Children playing football did not only have higher total amounts of daily PA, but also had higher amounts of PA during school time. During school time, children playing club football in their leisure time had 36% higher daily amount of PA and 43% higher PA at a vigorous level (both $p < 0.001$) than children participating in other club-sports.

The difference in amounts of PA between children playing football as their club sport and children doing other sport is larger during school time than total time. This may indicate that the higher activity levels among children playing club football is not only (or even mainly) due to high activity levels when participating in this leisure-time club activity, but also due to their higher levels of activity during school hours.

Compared to children not participating in club-sports, children doing other sports had higher daily amounts of vigorous activity ($p < 0.05$) but had neither significantly higher total daily minutes of moderate activity, nor higher likelihood of being active for an hour each day, nor higher amounts of activity during school time.

Activity levels during leisure-time club sports and school recess

Table 3 describes the activity levels during leisure-time club sports and during school recess. Children participating in club football did not have higher amounts of total or vigorous activity during the hours of their club-sports participation than children doing other types of club-sports, but did have higher amounts of moderate activity (28%, $p = 0.02$). However, during school breaks, children playing leisure-time club football had higher amounts of activity (46%, $p < 0.001$), (moderate (43%, $p < 0.001$) and vigorous (50%, $p = 0.004$)) than children doing other club-sports whereas children doing other club-sports did not have higher activity levels than children not doing any clubs sports.

Associations between playing club-football and daily PA when adjusted for gender

Since children's gender affects both their activity levels and the likelihood of playing club football, the above-described associations between club football participation and daily PA needs to be adjusted for gender. This was done using General Linear model. The results are described in Table 4. It can be seen that there is a gender-independent association between playing club football and the amount of PA in

Table 3. Activity levels of children: who played club football, participated in other club sports and undertook no leisure-time club sports.

	Played club football	Participated in other club sports	No club sports participation
Activity level during club sport			
% of time physically active	33.86 (18.32)	29.09 (13.44)	
% of time moderately active	18.93(10.64)[b]	14.77 (6.99)	
% of time vigorously active	14.94 (10.15)	14.32 (10.44)	
Activity level during school recess			
% of time physically active[aaa]	29.78 (11.37)[bbb]	20.44 (13.11)	19.87 (12.26)
% of time moderately active[aaa]	18.53 (6.31)[bbb]	12.95 (6.59)	13.31 (7.44)
% of time vigorously active[aaa]	11.25 (7.3)[bb]	7.48 (7.09)	6.56 (6.25)

Note: Data are presented as mean (SD).
[aaa]Difference between the three groups (ANOVA) is significant at $p < 0.001$.
[b]Difference between children who played football and children other sports significant at $p < 0.05$.
[bb]Difference between children who played football and children doing other sports significant at $p < 0.01$.
[bbb]Difference between children who played football and children doing other sports significant at $p < 0.001$.

Table 4. Associations between playing club football or not and measures of daily PA adjusted for gender.

		95% CI		
	B	Lower	Upper	p
Total activity (minutes of activity per day)	17.89	9.05	26.74	<0.001
School time activity (minutes of activity per day)	9.58	4.71	14.46	<0.001
Activity level during club sports (% of time physically active)	7.10%	1.23%	12.90%	0.018
Activity level during school recess (% of time physically active)	7.70%	3.78%	11.63%	<0.001

total, during school time, during clubs sports and during school recess. The interaction term of gender and playing football was not significantly associated to any of the PA measures, implying that the association between playing football and PA is not different for the two genders. This interaction term was therefore not included in any of the final models presented.

It is interesting to note that playing club football in free time has a strong association not only with total activity and activity levels during the sports time itself, but also with activity levels in school and school recess indicating that being more active during school recess is one of the main reasons children playing leisure-time club football are more active in total. To further support this hypotheses, Table 5 describes the association between playing club football and the total daily amount of activity when adjusted for activity levels during recess. It can be seen that adjusting for children's activity levels during recess decreases the higher amount of daily activity among club football players from $B = 17.89$ min/day to $B = 9.22$ min/day. This roughly indicates that almost half of club football's association to total daily activity stems from higher activity during school recess.

Discussion

According to modern sociological action theory,[18] human agency and hence children's physical activities can be regarded as a product of the interplay between local, social, cultural and material resources and the acting agent's (the child's) individual

Table 5. The association between playing club football and the daily amount of activity, when adjusting for gender and for activity levels during recess.

		95% CI		
	B	Low	High	p
Model 1: crude				
Playing football unadjusted (crude)	21.72	12.97	30.48	<0.001
Model 2: adjusting for gender				
Playing football	17.89	9.05	26.74	<0.001
Gender	9.70	4.87	14.54	<0.001
Model 3: adjusting for gender and recess PA level				
Playing football	9.22	1.44	16.99	0.020
Gender	3.61	−0.68	7.90	0.099
PA level during recess	112.68	95.74	129.61	<0.001

interests and abilities. Based on this understanding of PA as social practice, it can be hypothesized that in order to increase PA, the children's knowledge, skills and interest in a particular PA is crucial, but so too are the necessary material resources (sport and play facilities), social resources (others to play with) and cultural resources (rules, norms and values determining which activities are acceptable/'normal' for girls and boys to do in these settings).

In this study, children (most often boys) participating in club football during their leisure time had higher amounts of total daily PA resulting in a very high likelihood of being active more than the minimum recommended hour per day. This is in line with other more experimental studies which have shown very high activity levels when children play football.[19] However, an important contribution from this study is the observation that children participating in leisure-time club football were not only more active during this activity but also during school time in general, and school breaks in particular, than children doing other club-sports or no club-sports in their leisure time. This suggests that club football not only affects daily PA through the activity it creates in itself but is also an indicator of an interest in and an ability to play football which other studies have shown to be helpful resources for being active during recess in Danish schools.[20] In other words children's interest in and ability to play football affects their activities in other everyday contexts where there are opportunities to play this game. This is especially the case during school recess. As school recesses take up many weekly hours of children's lives, these abilities and interests have a great influence on the total amount of their activity.

On a more general level, the results suggest that the influence leisure-time club sport participation has on PA may differ as a result of the different PA levels of different sports, but also of how well the sport can be transferred to and played in other daily contexts for children's PA.

It might seem counterintuitive that the group of children participating in other leisure-time club sports than football did not have higher amounts of daily physical activity than the children not doing any club sports in their leisure time. It has been previously shown that[21] Danish children at the age 9–10 often have high activity levels in their daily contexts for self-organized outdoor play in which they spend many more hours each week and than the few hours per week typically spent participating in organized sport. In other words, at this age clubs sports participation per se is not a vital determinant of children's PA as those children who do not participate in sports[22] are often active elsewhere in other more self-organized ways. However, a club-football background seems to be an especially enabling resource for being physically active in these contexts.

Practical perspectives

The described association between football and the total daily amount of PA through high recess activity raises new questions about how best to use this knowledge to increase children's daily PA. In practice, trying to increase children's PA is often complex, as some of the patterns of inequality and stratification in PA practices are reflections of broader stratification mechanisms not easily changed by local PA initiatives alone.

Therefore, it remains hard to determine whether the solution to increase levels of PA lies in trying to make football a game for all during recess (for example by increasing the amount of playground space and facilities allocated to football and by trying to increase children's abilities and interest in playing football) or in trying to promote other easily self-organized physical activities in school recess and other informal play settings for children (for example by providing better facilities for these). Because the shaping of a child's interest in playing football rely on a wide range of socializing agents (families, peers, pedagogues, coaches, TV networks, etc.), it is not easily changed and considering also that children are different (not only across genders) with regard to their tastes, values, habits and skills, the last approach might be most effective from a public health intervention point of view and, importantly, more all-inclusive/democratic.

Limitations

A main limitation of this study is that it does not measure whether children are playing football during recess. However, other studies have shown how the football games at recess are dominated by 'football boys' who are very skilled and knowledgeable about football and who also play in clubs during their leisure time after school.[23]

As the data analysed is cross-sectional, it is hard to determine whether club football participation leads to high activity levels or whether children who are somehow disposed to be very physically active are more likely to choose this game as their club sport and school-ground activity. However, as sporting tastes are dependent on many social structural factors (such as the sporting interests of parents, friends, available sports-facilities in neighbourhood, etc.), the latter does not seem likely as a main explanation. Based on other studies of children's PA in Danish school grounds,[24] we interpret the association between club football and total PA and the mediating effect of school recess PA to be the result of football as a game that results in high activity levels when played and that Danish school grounds provide good facilities for football.

Conclusion

In the suburban Danish setting of this study, children playing club football as leisure-time club sport had higher total daily amounts of PA of both moderate and vigorous intensity than children doing other club-sports and children not doing club-sports. About half of the difference in total PA could be explained by higher activity levels during school recess alone.

The association between club football and total PA and the mediating effect of school recess PA can be interpreted to be the result of club football having high activity levels and of Danish school grounds offering good facilities for those who are able and interested to play football during the many hours of school recess each week.

On a more general level, the results indicate that the influence leisure-time club sport participation has on PA may differ according to different PA levels of different sports and also to how well the sport can be transferred to and played in other daily contexts for children's PA.

Disclosure statement

No potential conflict of interest was reported by the authors.

Notes

1. Andersen et al., 'Physical Activity and Clustered Cardiovascular Risk in Children: A Cross-sectional Study (The European Youth Heart Study)'; Dencker and Andersen, 'Health-related Aspects of Objectively Measured Daily Physical Activity in Children'; and Dencker and Andersen, 'Health-related Aspects of Objectively Measured Daily Physical Activity in Children', *Clinical Physiology and Functional Imaging* 28 (2008): 133–44.
2. Hansen, 'Hvorledes Idræt blev til folkesundhed'; World Health Organization, 'European Strategy for Child and Adolescent Health and Development'; and World Health Organization, 'The Origins and Evolution of Public Health'.
3. Jacobsen, *Idræt og velfærdspolitik* [Sport and welfare politics].
4. Basterfield et al., 'Longitudinal Associations between Sports Participation, Body Composition and Physical Activity from Childhood to Adolescence'; Nielsen et al., 'Predisposed to Participate? The Influence of Family Socio-economic Background on Children's Sports Participation and Daily Amount of Physical Activity'.
5. Nielsen et al., 'Predisposed to Participate? The Influence of Family Socio-economic Background on Children's Sports Participation and Daily Amount of Physical Activity'.
6. Laub, *Danskernes Motions- og Sportsvaner 2011*.
7. Ibid.
8. Bendiksen et al., 'Heart Rate Response and Fitness Effects of Various Types of Physical Education for 8- to 9-year-old Schoolchildren'; Randers et al., 'Effect of Game Format on Heart Rate, Activity Profile, and Player Involvement in Elite and Recreational Youth Players'; and Randers et al., 'Activity Profile and Physiological Response to Football Training for Untrained Males and Females, Elderly and Youngsters: Influence of the Number of Players'.
9. Pawlowski et al., '"Like a Football Camp for Boys". A Qualitative Exploration of Gendered Activity Patterns in Children's Self-organized Play during School Recess'; Pawlowski et al., 'Barriers for Recess Physical Activity: A Gender Specific Qualitative Focus Group Exploration'; Nielsen, Pfister, and Andersen, 'Gender Differences in the Daily Physical Activities of Danish School Children'; and Nielsen, *Children's Daily Physical Activity – Patterns and the Influence of Sociocultural Factors*.
10. Nielsen, *Children's Daily Physical Activity – Patterns and the Influence of Sociocultural Factors*.
11. Nielsen, Pfister, and Andersen, 'Gender Differences in the Daily Physical Activities of Danish School Children'; Nielsen, *Children's Daily Physical Activity – Patterns and the Influence of Sociocultural Factors*.
12. Ekelund et al., 'Physical Activity Assessed by Activity Monitor and Doubly Labelled Water in Children'.
13. De Vries et al., 'Clinimetric Review of Motion Sensors in Children and Adolescents'; Brage et al., 'Reexamination of Validity and Reliability of the CSA Monitor in Walking and Running'; and Mattocks et al., 'Early Life Determinants of Physical Activity in 11 to 12 year Olds'.
14. Eiberg et al., 'Maximum Oxygen Uptake and Objectively Measured Physical Activity in Danish Children 6–7 Years of Age: The Copenhagen School Child Intervention Study'; Dencker et al., 'Daily Physical Activity in Swedish Children Aged 8–11 Years'.
15. The group with three days of measurement and the group with four days of measurement did not differ in their average amounts of daily activity.
16. Trost et al., 'Validity of the Computer Science and Applications (CSA) Activity Monitor in Children'; Puyau et al., 'Validation and Calibration of Physical Activity Monitors in Children'; Treuth et al., 'Defining Accelerometer Thresholds for Activity Intensities in Adolescent Girls'; Sirard et al., 'Calibration and Evaluation of an Objective Measure of Physical Activity in Preschool Children'; and Mattocks et al., 'Calibration of an Accelerometer during Free-living Activities in Children'.
17. Strong et al., 'Evidence Based Physical Activity for School-age Youth'.
18. Bourdieu, *The Logic of Practice*; Giddens, *The Constitution of Society – Outline of the Theory of Structuration*.
19. Bendiksen et al., 'Heart Rate Response and Fitness Effects of Various Types of Physical Education for 8- to 9-year-old Schoolchildren'; Randers et al., 'Effect of Game Format

on Heart Rate, Activity Profile, and Player Involvement in Elite and Recreational Youth Players'.
20. Pawlowski et al., '"Like a Football Camp for Boys". A Qualitative Exploration of Gendered Activity Patterns in Children's Self-organized Play during School Recess'.
21. Nielsen, *Children's Daily Physical Activity – Patterns and the Influence of Sociocultural Factors*.
22. Often children of Low SEP and/or ethnic minority background Nielsen et al., 'Predisposed to Participate? The Influence of Family Socio-economic Background on Children's Sports Participation and Daily Amount of Physical Activity'; Nielsen, *Children's Daily Physical Activity – Patterns and the Influence of Sociocultural Factors*.
23. Pawlowski et al., '"Like a Football Camp for Boys". A Qualitative Exploration of Gendered Activity Patterns in Children's Self-organized Play during School Recess'.
24. Ibid.; Nielsen et al., 'School Playground Facilities as a Determinant of Children's Daily Activity – A Cross-sectional Study of Danish Primary School Children'.

References

Andersen, L.B., M. Harro, L.B. Sardinha, K. Froberg, U. Ekelund, S. Brage, and S. Anderssen. 'Physical Activity and Clustered Cardiovascular Risk in Children: A Cross-sectional Study (The European Youth Heart Study)'. *The Lancet* 368, no. 9532 (2006): 299–304.

Anderson, S. *Civil Sociality – Children, Sport and Cultural Policy in Denmark*. Charlotte, NC: Information Age Publishing, 2008.

Basterfield, L., J.K. Reilly, M.S. Pearce, K.N. Parkinson, A.J. Adamson, J.J. Reilly, and S.A. Vella. 'Longitudinal Associations between Sports Participation, Body Composition and Physical Activity from Childhood to Adolescence'. *Journal of Science and Medicine in Sport* 18 (2015): 178–82.

Bendiksen, M., C.A. Williams, T. Hornstrup, H. Clausen, J. Kloppenborg, D. Shumikhin, J. Brito et al. 'Heart Rate Response and Fitness Effects of Various Types of Physical Education for 8- to 9-year-old Schoolchildren'. *European Journal of Sport Science*, 14 (2014): 861–9.

Bourdieu, P. *The Logic of Practice*. Cambridge: Polity Press, 1997.

Brage, S., N. Wedderkopp, P.W. Franks, L. Bo Andersen, and K. Froberg. 'Reexamination of Validity and Reliability of the CSA Monitor in Walking and Running'. *Medicine & Science in Sports & Exercise* 35, no. 8 (2003): 1447–54.

Dencker, M., and L.B. Andersen. 'Health-related Aspects of Objectively Measured Daily Physical Activity in Children'. *Clinical Physiology and Functional Imaging* 28, no. 3 (2008): 133–44.

Dencker, M., O. Thorsson, M.K. Karlsson, C. Linden, J. Svensson, P. Wollmer, and L.B. Andersen. 'Daily Physical Activity in Swedish Children Aged 8–11 Years'. *Scandinavian Journal of Medicine and Science in Sports* 16, no. 4 (2006): 252–7.

De Vries, S.I., I. Bakker, M. Hopman-Rock, R. Hirasing, and W. van Mechelen. 'Clinimetric Review of Motion Sensors in Children and Adolescents'. *Journal of Clinical Epidemiology* 59, no. 7 (2006): 670–80.

Eiberg, S., H. Hasselstrom, V. Gronfeldt, K. Froberg, J. Svensson, and L.B. Andersen. 'Maximum Oxygen Uptake and Objectively Measured Physical Activity in Danish Children 6–7 Years of Age: The Copenhagen School Child Intervention Study'. *British Journal of Sports Medicine* 39, no. 10 (2005): 725–30.

Ekelund, U., M. Sjostrom, A. Yngve, E. Poortvliet, A. Nilsson, K. Froberg, N. Wedderkopp, and K. Westerterp. 'Physical Activity Assessed by Activity Monitor and Doubly Labelled Water in Children'. *Medicine & Science in Sports & Exercise* 33, no. 2 (2001): 275–81.

Giddens, A. *The Constitution of Society – Outline of the Theory of Structuration*. London: Polity Press, 1984.

Hansen, J. 'Hvorledes Idræt blev til folkesundhed'. [How sport and exercise became public health]. *Forum for Idræt* 26, no. 2 (2010): 9–20.

Horne, J., A. Tomlinson, and G. Whannel. 'Socialisation – Social Interaction and Development'. In *Understanding Sport*, ed. John Horne, Allan Tomlinson, and Garry Whannel, 129–55. London: Spon Press, 1999.

Ibsen, B., and L. Ottesen. 'Foreninger som læringsrum for demokrati og sundhed'. [Associations and clubs as settings for learning about democracy and health]. In *Voksnes læringsrum*, ed. Carsten Nejst Jensen, 413–31. Værløse: Billesø og Baltzer, 2005.

Jacobsen, P.J., L. Ottesen, A.B. Grønkjær, B.V. Madsen, A.M. La Cour, and C. Østergaard, eds. 'Idræt og velfærdspolitik'. [Sport and welfare politics]. Special issue *Forum for Idræt* 27, no. 1 (2011): 65–89.

Kjønniksen, L., N. Anderssen, and B. Wold. 'Organized Youth Sport as a Predictor of Physical Activity in Adulthood'. *Scandinavian Journal of Medicine & Science in Sports* 19, no. 5 (2009): 646–54.

Korsgaard, O. *Kampen om kroppen* [The struggle about the body]. København: Gyldendal, 1997.

Laub, T.B. *Danskernes Motions- og Sportsvaner 2011* [Exercise and sports participation in Denmark 2011]. København: IDAN, 2013.

Mattocks, C., S. Leary, A. Ness, K. Deere, J. Saunders, K. Tilling, and J. Kirkby. 'Calibration of an Accelerometer during Free-living Activities in Children'. *International Journal of Pediatric Obesity* 2, no. 4 (2007): 218–26.

Mattocks, C., A. Ness, K. Deere, K. Tilling, S. Leary, S.N. Blair, and C. Riddoch. 'Early Life Determinants of Physical Activity in 11 to 12 Year Olds: Cohort Study'. *BMJ* 336, no. 7634 (2008): 26–9.

Nielsen, G. 'Children's Daily Physical Activity – Patterns and the Influence of Sociocultural Factors'. PhD thesis, Department of Exercise and Sport Sciences, University of Copenhagen, 2011.

Nielsen, G., A. Bugge, B. Hermansen, J. Svensson, and L.B. Andersen. 'School Playground Facilities as a Determinant of Children's Daily Activity – A Cross-sectional Study of Danish Primary School Children'. *Journal of Physical Activity and Health* 9, no. 1 (2012): 104–14.

Nielsen, G., V. Grønfeldt, J. Toftegaard-Støckel, and L.B. Andersen. 'Predisposed to Participate? The Influence of Family Socio-economic Background on Children's Sports Participation and Daily Amount of Physical Activity'. *Sport in Society* 15, no. 1 (2012): 1–27.

Nielsen, G., G. Pfister, and L.B. Bo Andersen. 'Gender Differences in the Daily Physical Activities of Danish School Children'. *European Physical Education Review* 17, no. 1 (2011): 69–90.

Ottesen, L., and O. Skjerk. *Inaktivitetsundersøgelse: Sammenfatning* [The inactivity study]. København: Institut for Idræt, Københavns Universitet, 2006.

Pawlowski, C.S., C. Ergler, T. Tjørnhøj-Thomsen, J. Schipperijn, and J. Troelsen. 'Barriers for Recess Physical Activity: A Gender Specific Qualitative Focus Group Exploration'. *BMC Public Health* 14, no. 1 (2014): 639.

Pawlowski, C.S., C. Ergler, T. Tjørnhøj-Thomsen, J. Schipperijn, and J. Troelsen. '"Like a Soccer Camp for Boys". A Qualitative Exploration of Gendered Activity Patterns in Children's Self-organized Play during School Recess'. *European Physical Education Review* 12 (2014): 1–17.

Pestoff, V.A. 'Making Citizenship Meaningful in the Twenty-first Century'. In *A Democratic Architecture for the Welfare State*, ed. Victor Alexis Pestoff, 1–20. Oxon: Routledge, 2009.

Puyau, M.R., A.L. Adolph, F.A. Vohra, and N.F. Butte. 'Validation and Calibration of Physical Activity Monitors in Children'. *Obesity Research* 10, no. 3 (2002): 150–7.

Randers, M.B., T.B. Andersen, L.S. Rasmussen, M.N. Larsen, and P. Krustrup. 'Effect of Game Format on Heart Rate, Activity Profile, and Player Involvement in Elite and Recreational Youth Players'. *Scandinavian Journal of Medicine & Science in Sports* 24, suppl. 1 (2014): 17–26.

Randers, M.B., L. Nybo, J. Petersen, J.J. Nielsen, L. Christiansen, M. Bendiksen, J. Brito, J. Bangsbo, and P. Krustrup. 'Activity Profile and Physiological Response to Football Training for Untrained Males and Females, Elderly and Youngsters: Influence of the Number of Players'. *Scandinavian Journal of Medicine & Science in Sports* 20, suppl. 1 (2010): 14–23.

Sirard, J.R., S.G. Trost, M. Pfeiffer, M. Dowda, and R.P. Pate. 'Calibration and Evaluation of an Objective Measure of Physical Activity in Preschool Children'. *Journal of Physical Activity & Health* 2, no. 3 (2005): 345–57.

Strong, W.B., R.M. Malina, C.J. Blimkie, S.R. Daniels, R.K. Dishman, B. Gutin, and Albert C. Hergenroeder. 'Evidence Based Physical Activity for School-age Youth'. *The Journal of Pediatrics* 146, no. 6 (2005): 732–7.

Treuth, M.S., K. Schmitz, D.J. Catellier, R.G. McMurray, D.M. Murray, M.J. Almeida, S. Going, J.E. Norman, and R. Pate. 'Defining Accelerometer Thresholds for Activity Intensities in Adolescent Girls'. *Medicine & Science in Sports & Exercise* 36, no. 7 (2004): 1259–66.

Trost, S.G., D.S. Ward, S.M. Moorehead, P.D. Watson, W. Riner, and J.R. Burke. 'Validity of the Computer Science and Applications (CSA) Activity Monitor in Children'. *Medicine & Science in Sports & Exercise* 30, no. 4 (1998): 629–33.

World Health Organization. *The Origins and Evolution of Public Health; in WHO: New Challenges for Public Health*. Geneva: WHO, 1996.

World Health Organization Europe. *European Strategy for Child and Adolescent Health and Development*. Copenhagen: The WHO Regional Office for Europe, 2005.

Football for health: getting strategic

Simon Lansley[a] and Daniel Parnell[a,b]

[a]ConnectSport UK Ltd, London, UK; [b]Centre for Active Lifestyles, Institute of Sport, Physical Activity and Leisure, Leeds Beckett University, Leeds, UK

Community foundations and charities operating within professional football clubs are being championed as a vehicle to deliver on the Public Health agenda. This personal commentary from the authors offers insight into the context of football for health drawing on the relevant research literature and their experiences working within the football industry in England. The football and health examples highlight under-resourced and under-evaluated interventions, whilst highlighting the importance of partnership working. The authors hope to support those in football and health in getting strategic through their interventions, evaluations and partnerships, in order to capitalize the potential of football in supporting the objectives of Public Health England.

Football has been the go to sport for not only the sport for development movement, but also for corporate enterprises wishing to deliver on a corporate social responsibility (CSR) agenda.[1] Community foundations of professional football clubs have been ushered to the front of the queue by big brands, business and clubs alike to deliver on social welfare objectives, including physical activity and health.[2] It is time for community foundations and charities operating within professional football clubs to step out of the shadows and start to shout about their impact and celebrate their value. This personal commentary from the authors offers insight into the context of football for health drawing on the relevant research literature and their experiences working within the football industry in England. The authors seek to offer those working within football for health a clarion call get strategic through their interventions, evaluations, and partnerships, in order to capitalize their potential and support the objectives of Public Health England.

The socio-political and economic context provides an interesting era of policy and in turn opportunity for community foundations to recruit additional resources to tackle the health agenda.[3] For those who have got the money, CSR still does not feature high on the list of business priorities. Indeed, many CSR initiatives still unable to reconcile the incongruence between short-term business objectives and longer-term social welfare issues.[4] Football clubs must of course focus on TV revenue, sponsorships deals or season ticket sales, while national governing bodies find their time taken up worrying about how to hit participation targets[5] or managing one public relations crisis after another.[6] Plus, at the top end of sport it's an intoxicating business; egos and reputations can grow so big they sometimes seem to have lost touch with the real world.[7] Senior executives still talk about their organizations 'giving away' money to community projects, as if it they were born of altruism.[8]

It is this intersection between the commercially oriented glitz and glamour of professional football clubs and the never-ending quest for increased participation (amongst other social issues) that you will find the average football club community foundation. Most of these organizations are lucky to make the any other business on the agenda at the Board meeting often because the concept of SROI (Social Return on Investment) is still in its infancy within football and cost-effectiveness is either beyond either the evaluation skill base of practitioners or the budget constraints of community foundations [or both].[9] Even if those working within a club's community foundation engage with the local populace more than anyone else at the club, it is just so damned hard to measure this engagement in monetary terms to a CEO (chief executive officer) and broader stakeholders.[10]

Football club community foundations have been caught up in a period of exponential growth through increased resource availability and funding opportunities from the days of the then Labour government in 1997.[11] Alongside this, project delivery has become more complex as delivery agendas have shifted from traditional football coaching in schools to new areas such as health improvement.[12] Community foundations are now at a new juncture, were their departments, in many cases have grown in size, and directors have, and still are chasing funding resources to now sustain their organizations. Previously, it has been highlighted that in times of austerity, inflated promises – often through programme targets – can be made.[13] This has been observed by the authors in a variety of football and health improvement contexts, which has prompted this personal insight article. The authors highlight and describe two personal experiences in the following section. Using these two examples, the authors illustrate some of the contextual and applied challenges faced by practitioners in this current era of football and health.

In the first example, funding has been provided to football club community foundation to deliver a new area of work in football health improvement. This involved the community foundation delivering a 10-month football programme for participants with mental health issues on a budget of £10,000 without consideration of process or impact evaluation. This was not only a new area of work for the community foundation [i.e. working with participants with mental health issues], but also an agenda the current staff had little or no experience or any requisite skill for delivering. The second example concerned the provision of funding totalling £20,000 to a community foundation, by a local Public Health commissioner. To receive the funding the community foundation had to agree to ensure 2000 men lose a clinically significant amount of weight (i.e. a 5% reduction in weight) within at 12 months. These are not isolated cases, just two examples to underline the authors growing concern within the industry.

To the authors, both these cases (and projects) are under-resourced and supported. In order to approach a new avenue of work, you would expect project staff to require a new skill base and expertise.[14] Further both cases highlight an absence of evaluation requirement beyond the measurement of participant weight pre-and post-programme in the latter case. Given that guidance supports evaluation costs at between 10 and 20% of programme budgets,[15] it is clear that these examples lack appropriate support and funding and potentially place community foundation managers and practitioners into potentially unethical situations commissioners [and/or investors], whereby they are driven towards inflating programme targets. The authors have experienced similar cases on scaled up and scaled down versions of the two examples provided, and they believe such experiences will resonate with many reading this article from both health promotion and sport for health backgrounds. The authors hope those readers would agree that these programmes should not be funded through this approach. Further, the authors call for a strategic approach to programme funding and evaluation, which includes developing both delivery and evaluation partnerships, and the provision of adequate and relevant support, which includes committing to realistic resources and outcomes.[16]

For football club community foundations to become financially viable and work towards sustainability, they need to become more focused, strategic and adopt sound business planning. That means defining a product (or service) and its value simply and clearly, ensuring there is a good, healthy market for that product. For football and health, this could be led by national, regional, and/or local needs. It might be for any group across the lifespan, from children through to older adults. Health or social issues, such as, inactivity, obesity, heart disease, smoking cessation, alcohol consumption or homelessness, could initiate this need. Indeed, Public Health England endorses a national needs assessment, which provides a 'big picture' for health priorities, which must be dovetailed with local priorities and perspectives.[17] Whatever the need, football club community foundations must focus on these strategic objectives. This will help them avoid getting side-tracked, often on programmes set up to fail by commissioners or investors seeking unrealistic targets. This will mean community foundations must be able and strategic enough to say 'no' to so-called opportunities, which fall outside this strategic need and subsequent focus. From the authors applied experiences, the community foundations that will prosper during this complex socio-economic and political time are those which are run on strict business grounds, focused on evidencing impact, using where feasible SROI and cost-effectiveness, whilst remaining mindful of their profit and loss. For community foundations, the message is clear: be strategic; strategic with their intervention and subsequent evaluation.

So what do we know about football and health? Football has been used to deliver health interventions[18] across a range of groups across the lifespan (i.e. children to older people) whom exhibit a range of diseases and conditions.[19] Football clubs can engage large numbers supporter and people within their local communities, as such interventions have attempted to capitalize on this link to improve people's health.[20] Football club-based interventions have been shown to improve lifestyle behaviours, such as physical activity, diet, smoking and alcohol consumption in men and older men,[21] the management of weight and BMI in men and women[22] and improved mental well-being in men.[23] Moreover, football has been found to be an important factor for engaging children in fun and enjoyable physical activity,[24] for engaging families in positive lifestyle changes[25] and supporting positive opportunities for older adults to engage in physical and social activities.[26] Importantly, football clubs (through community foundations) are able to attract diverse groups from the community on to health improvement interventions.[27]

The growing evidence base supporting the role of football in health improvement is extremely valuable for community foundations. Yet, as Public Health England endeavour to protect and improve the nation's health and well-being, and reduce inequalities, they will seek effective interventions that can evidence value for money.[28] One intervention, which has been, able to offer an exemplar evaluation to support the case of football health improvement is 'Football Fans in Training'

(FFIT), a gender-sensitized, weight-management intervention delivered across 13 Scottish Premier League football clubs.[29] This was a pragmatic randomized control trial of $N = 747$ men aged 35–65 years old with a BMI of 28 kg/m^2 or higher. After one year, the mean difference in weight loss between the intervention and control groups – adjusted for baseline weight and club – was 4.94 kg, whilst percentage weight loss was 4.36%. Not only was FFIT efficacious, but also it was also cost-effective.

Quality-adjusted life year (QALYs) is a measure of the state of health of a person or group in which the benefits, in terms of length of life, are adjusted to reflect the quality of life. One QALY is equal to 1 year of life in perfect health. QALYs are calculated by estimating the years of life remaining for a participant following an intervention and weighting each year with a quality of life score (on a 0 to 1 scale). This can be measured in terms of the person's ability to perform the activities of daily life, freedom from pain, and mental disturbance.[30] Results from FFIT indicated that the cost per QALY gained fell below the threshold of £20,000 used by NICE, and in turn, the intervention was considered cost-effective. Overall, the FFIT programme enabled a substantial proportion of men to lose a clinically important amount of weight. FFIT is a powerful piece of research that should be used by other community foundations. However, given the costs of FFIT [in the region of £1 million], it is unlikely that community foundations could resource this level of research. As such community foundations should seek to learn from this research and develop workable programmes and evaluations in their setting.

During this period of economic austerity, it will be those who can evidence their impact that are able to develop and sustain their organization and impact.[31] No matter the size of a football club community foundation's turnover, it is apparent that they must work towards being able to provide evidence of their impact, through the development and delivery of evidence-based interventions, alongside easy-to-define outcomes and precise M&E (monitoring and evaluation), which will be imperative to commissioners and investors. As such, this may also involve recruiting an independent project partner (such as a local university) to provide support and guidance for evidenced-based practice, project planning and research and evaluation.[32] For the latter, it will be important for research and evaluations to be both strategic and aligned with the resources of the community foundations in the current economic climate.

In summary, the potential of health improvement delivered through community foundations has some evidence of effectiveness. This will be a potent resource for community foundations preparing to embark on football and health improvement to inform their interventions. It is critical to utilize this evidence into intervention planning and in turn to develop relevant evaluation measures, through partnerships and then share findings with potential commissioners and investors. Football offers a very attractive and potential powerful vehicle for health improvement. For us to truly value the role community foundations to support Public Health England, it is time for them to get strategic with their interventions, evaluations and partnerships.

Disclosure statement

No potential conflict of interest was reported by the authors.

Notes

1. Doane, 'The Myth of CSR'; Slack and Shrives, 'Beyond the Game. Perceptions and Practices of Corporate Social Responsibility in the Professional Sport Industry'; Coalter, 'Sport-in-Development: Development for and through Sport?' 48; Levermore, 'The Paucity of, and Dilemma in, Evaluating Corporate Social Responsibility for Development through Sport'.
2. Quazi, 'Identifying the Determinants of Corporate Managers' Perceived Social Obligations'; Smith and Westerbeek, 'Sport as a Vehicle for Deploying Corporate Social Responsibility'; Babiak and Wolfe, 'Determinants of Corporate Social Responsibility in Professional Sport: Internal and External Factors'; Hamil and Morrow, 'Corporate Social Responsibility in the Scottish Premier League. Context and Motivation'; Parnell et al., 'Football in the Community Schemes: Exploring the Effectiveness of an Intervention in Promoting Positive Healthful Behaviour Change'; Parnell and Richardson, 'Introduction: Football and Inclusivity'.
3. Parnell, Millward, and Spracklen, 'Sport and Austerity in the UK: An Insight into Liverpool 2014'.
4. Newell, 'Citizenship, Accountability and Community. The Limits of CSR Agenda'.
5. SkySports, *Sport England Slash Netball Funding*; Gibson, *Sport England's £1.6 m Cut to the FA 'a Warning over Grassroots Failure'*.
6. BBC, *Greg Dyke: FA Chairman Says Grassroots Football 'in Crisis'*.
7. Parnell et al., 'Implementing "Monitoring and Evaluation" Techniques within a Premier League Football in the Community Scheme'.
8. Bishop, 'Funding Football from the Grassroots to the Championship', Research paper on behalf of the All Party Football Group, 13.
9. King, *Local Authority Sport and Recreation Services in England: Where Next? The Association for Public Service Excellence*; Parnell et al., 'Football in the Community Schemes: Exploring the Effectiveness of an Intervention in Promoting Positive Healthful Behaviour Change'; Hunt et al., 'A Gender-sensitised Weight Loss and Healthy Living Programme for Overweight and Obese Men Delivered by Scottish Premier League Football Clubs (FFIT): A Pragmatic Randomised Controlled Trial'.
10. McGuire and Fenoglio, 'Football in the Community: Resources and Opportunities'; Karnani, 'The Case Against Corporate Social Responsibility'; Parnell et al., 'Football in the Community Schemes: Exploring the Effectiveness of an Intervention in Promoting Positive Healthful Behaviour Change'.
11. Coalter, *A Wider Social Role for Sport: Who's Keeping the Score?*
12. Parnell et al., 'Football in the Community Schemes: Exploring the Effectiveness of an Intervention in Promoting Positive Healthful Behaviour Change'.
13. Weiss, 'Where Politics and Evaluation Research Meet'.
14. Parnell et al., 'Football in the Community Schemes: Exploring the Effectiveness of an Intervention in Promoting Positive Healthful Behaviour Change'.
15. Dugdill and Stratton, *Evaluating Sport and Physical Activity Interventions: A Guide for Practitioners*.
16. Pringle et al., 'Assessing the Impact of Football-based Health Improvement Programmes: Stay Onside, Avoid Own Goals and Score with the Evaluation!'.
17. Public Health England, *Our Priorities for 2013/14*.
18. Parnell et al., 'Football in the Community Schemes: Exploring the Effectiveness of an Intervention in Promoting Positive Healthful Behaviour Change'.
19. The Premier League, 'Premier League Investing to Support PE and Sports in Primary School'; Parnell and Richardson, 'Introduction: Football and Inclusivity'.
20. Pringle and Sayer, 'It's a Goal!: Basing a Community Psychiatric Nursing Service in a Local Football Stadium'; Brady et al., 'Sustained Benefits of a Health Project for Middle Aged Football Supporters at Glasgow Celtic and Rangers Football Clubs'; Parnell et al., 'Football in the Community Schemes: Exploring the Effectiveness of an Intervention in Promoting Positive Healthful Behaviour Change'; Pringle et al., 'Effect of a Health-improvement Pilot Programme for Older Adults Delivered by a Professional Football Club: The Burton Albion Case Study'.
21. Pringle et al., 'Health Improvement for Men and Hard-to-engage-men Delivered in English Premier League Football Clubs'; Bingham et al., 'Fit Fans: Perspectives of a

Practitioner and Understanding Participant Health Needs within a Health Promotion Programme for Older Men Delivered within an English Premier League Football Club'.

22. Hunt et al., 'A Gender-sensitised Weight Loss and Healthy Living Programme for Overweight and Obese Men Delivered by Scottish Premier League Football Clubs (FFIT): A Pragmatic Randomised Controlled Trial'; Rutherford et al., '"Motivate": The Effect of a Football in the Community Delivered Weight Loss Programme on over 35-year old Men and Women's Cardiovascular Risk Factors'.
23. Pringle and Sayer, 'It's a Goal!: Basing a Community Psychiatric Nursing Service in a Local Football Stadium'.
24. Parnell et al., 'Football in the Community Schemes: Exploring the Effectiveness of an Intervention in Promoting Positive Healthful Behaviour Change'.
25. Curran et al., 'Ethnographic Engagement from within a Football in the Community Programme at an English Premier League Football Club'.
26. Parnell et al., 'Reaching Older People with Physical Activity Delivered in Football Clubs: The Reach, Adoption and Implementation Characteristics of the Extra Time Programme'.
27. Parnell and Richardson, 'Introduction: Football and Inclusivity'; Zwolinsky et al., 'Re: World Cup 2014: Festival of Football or Alcohol?'
28. Public Health England, *Our Priorities for 2013/14.*
29. Hunt et al., 'A Gender-sensitised Weight Loss and Healthy Living Programme for Overweight and Obese Men Delivered by Scottish Premier League Football Clubs (FFIT): A Pragmatic Randomised Controlled Trial'.
30. NICE, *Measuring Effectiveness and Cost Effectiveness: The QALY.*
31. Zwolinsky, S., 'Re: World Cup 2014: Festival of Football or Alcohol?'; Parnell et al., 'Comments on Bruun, D.M. *et al.* Community-Based Recreational Football: A Novel Approach to Promote Physical Activity and Quality of Life in Prostate Cancer Survivors. *Int. J. Environ. Res. Public Health* 2014, 11, 5557–5585—Time to Raise Our Game'.
32. Pringle et al., 'Assessing the Impact of Football-based Health Improvement Programmes: Stay Onside, Avoid Own Goals and Score with the Evaluation!'; Parnell et al., 'Understanding Football as a Vehicle for Enhancing Social Inclusion: Using an Intervention Mapping Framework'; Parnell et al., 'Implementing "Monitoring and Evaluation" Techniques within a Premier League Football in the Community Scheme'.

References

Babiak, K., and R. Wolfe. 'Determinants of Corporate Social Responsibility in Professional Sport: Internal and External Factors'. *Journal of Sport Management* 23 (2009): 717–42.
BBC. *Greg Dyke: FA Chairman says grassroots football 'in crisis'.* 2014. http://www.bbc.co.uk/sport/0/football/29575890 (accessed December 10, 2014).
Bingham, D.D., D. Parnell, K. Curran, R. Jones, and D. Richardson. 'Fit Fans: Perspectives of a Practitioner and Understanding Participant Health Needs within a Health Promotion Programme for Older Men Delivered within an English Premier League Football Club'. *Soccer & Society* 15, no. 6 (2014): 883–901.
Bishop, D., J. Breeze, S. Danczuk, and G. Bailey. 'Funding Football from the Grassroots to the Championship.' Research Paper on Behalf of the All Party Football Group, Manchester, 2014.
Coalter, Fred. *A Wider Social Role for Sport: Who's Keeping the Score?* London: Routledge, 2007.
Coalter, F. 'Sport-in-Development: Development for and through Sport?' In *Sport and Social Capital*, ed. M. Nicholson and R. Hoye, 39–67. Oxford: Elsevier Butterworth-Heinemann, 2008.
Curran, K., D.D. Bingham, D. Richardson, and D. Parnell. 'Ethnographic Engagement from within a Football in the Community Programme at an English Premier League Football Club'. *Soccer & Society* 15, no. 6 (2014): 934–50.
Doane, D. 'The Myth of CSR'. *Stanford Social Innovation Review* (2005): 23–9. http://ssir.org/pdf/2005FA_Feature_Doane.pdf

Dugdill, L., and G. Stratton. *Evaluating Sport and Physical Activity Interventions: A Guide for Practitioners*. University of Salford, 2013. http://usir.salford.ac.uk/3148/1/Dugdill_and_Stratton_2007.pdf (accessed September 24, 2013).

Gibson, O. *Sport England's £1.6 m Cut to the FA 'A Warning over Grassroots Failure'*. 2014. http://www.theguardian.com/football/2014/mar/27/sport-england-funding-cut-fa-warning-grassroots-golf-netball-hockey-rowing (accessed December 10, 2014).

Hamil, S., and S. Morrow. 'Corporate Social Responsibility in the Scottish Premier League: Context and Motivation'. *European Sport Management Quarterly* 11, no. 2 (2011): 143–70.

Hunt, K., S. Wyke, C.M. Gray, A.S. Anderson, A. Brady, C. Bunn, P.T. Donnon et al. 'A Gender-sensitised Weight Loss and Healthy Living Programme for Overweight and Obese Men Delivered by Scottish Premier League Football Clubs (FFIT): A Pragmatic Randomised Controlled Trial'. *The Lancet* 383 (2014): 1211–21. doi:10.1016/S0140-6736(13)62420-4.

Karnani, A. 'The Case against Corporate Social Responsibility'. *The Wall Street Journal* (2014). http://online.wsj.com/news/articles/SB10001424052748703338004575230112664504890?mg=reno64-wsj&url=http%3A%2F%2Fonline.wsj.com%2Farticle%2FSB100014240527487033380045752301126645048904890.html (accessed December 10, 2014).

King, N. *Local Authority Sport and Recreation Services in England: Where Next?* The Association for Public Service Excellence, 2012. http://www.apse.org.uk/apse/index.cfm/research/current-research-programme/local-authority-sport-and-recreation-services-in-england-where-next/local-authority-sport-and-recreation-services-in-england-where-next/ (accessed December 10, 2014).

Levermore, R. 'The Paucity of, and Dilemma in, Evaluating Corporate Social Responsibility for Development through Sport'. *Third World Quarterly* 32, no. 3 (2011): 551–69.

McGuire, B., and R. Fenoglio. *Football in the Community: Resources and Opportunities*. Manchester: Manchester Metropolitan University, Department of Exercise and Sport Science, 2004.

National Institute for Health and Care Excellence. *Measuring Effectiveness and Cost Effectiveness: The QALY*. NICE, 2010. https://www.nice.org.uk/proxy/?sourceurl=http://www.nice.org.uk/newsroom/features/measuringeffectivenessandcosteffectivenesstheqaly.jsp (accessed December 14, 2014).

Newell, P. 'Citizenship, Accountability and Community: The Limits of the CSR Agenda'. *International Affairs* 81, no. 3 (2005): 541–57.

Parnell, D., P. Millward, and K. Spracklen. 'Sport and Austerity in the UK: An Insight into Liverpool 2014'. *Journal of Policy Research in Tourism, Leisure and Events* 7 (2014): 200–203. doi:10.1080/19407963.2014.968309.

Parnell, D., A. Pringle, J. McKenna, and S. Zwolinsky. 'Comments on Bruun, D.M. *et al.* Community-Based Recreational Football: A Novel Approach to Promote Physical Activity and Quality of Life in Prostate Cancer Survivors. *Int. J. Environ. Res. Public Health* 2014, 11, 5557–5585—Time to Raise Our Game'. *International Journal of Environmental Research and Public Health* 11, no. 7 (2014): 6842–3.

Parnell, D., A. Pringle, P. Widdop, and S. Zwolinsky. 'Understanding Football as a Vehicle for Enhancing Social Inclusion: Using an Intervention Mapping Framework'. *Social Inclusion* 3 7, no. 2 (2015): 200–3.

Parnell, D., A. Pringle, S. Zwolinsky, J. McKenna, Z. Rutherford, D. Richardson, L. Trotter, M. Rigby, and M.J. Hargreaves. 'Reaching Older People with Physical Activity Delivered in Football Clubs: The Reach, Adoption and Implementation Characteristics of the Extra Time Programme'. *BMC Public Health* 15 (2015). doi: 10.1186/s12889-015-1560-5. http://www.biomedcentral.com/1471-2458/15/220

Parnell, D., and D. Richardson. 'Introduction: Football and Inclusivity'. *Soccer & Society* 15, no. 6 (2014): 823–7.

Parnell, D., G. Stratton, B. Drust, and D. Richardson. 'Football in the Community Schemes: Exploring the Effectiveness of an Intervention in Promoting Healthful Behaviour Change'. *Soccer & Society* 14 (2013): 35–51.

Parnell, D., G. Stratton, B. Drust, and D. Richardson. 'Implementing "Monitoring and Evaluation" Techniques within a Premier League Football in the Community Scheme'. In

Routledge Handbook of Sport and Social Responsibility, ed. Juan Luis Paramio Salcines, Kathy Babiak, and Geoff Walters, 328–43. London: Routledge, 2013.

Pringle, A., J. Hargreaves, L. Lozano, J. McKenna, and S. Zwolinsky. 'Assessing the Impact of Football-Based Health Improvement Programmes: Stay Onside, Avoid Own Goals and Score with the Evaluation!'. *Soccer & Society* 15, no. 6 (2014): 970–87.

Pringle, A., D. Parnell, S. Zwolinsky, J. Hargreaves, and J. McKenna. 'Effect of a Health-improvement Pilot Programme for Older Adults Delivered by a Professional Football Club: The Burton Albion Case Study'. *Soccer & Society* 15 (2014): 902–18.

Pringle, A., and P. Sayers. 'It's a Goal!: Basing a Community Psychiatric Nursing Service in a Local Football Stadium'. *The Journal of the Royal Society for the Promotion of Health* 124 (2006): 234–8.

Pringle. A., S. Zwolinsky, J. McKenna, S. Robertson, A. Daly-Smith, and A. White. 'Health Improvement for Men and Hard-to-Engage-Men Delivered in English Premier League Football Clubs'. *Health Education Research* 29 (2014): 503–20.

Public Health England. *Our Priorities for 2013/14.* Public Health England, 2013. https://www.gov.uk/government/uploads/system/uploads/attachment_data/file/192676/Our_priorities_final.pdf (accessed January 10, 2015).

Quazi, A.M. 'Identifying the Determinants of Corporate Managers' Perceived Social Obligations'. *Management Decision* 41, no. 9 (2003): 822–31.

Rutherford, Z., and B. Gough, S. Seymour-Smith, C R Matthews, J. Wilcox, D. Parnell, and A. Pringle. '"Motivate": The Effect of a Football in the Community Delivered Weight Loss Programme on over 35-Year Old Men and Women's Cardiovascular Risk Factors'. *Soccer & Society* 15, no. 6 (2014): 951–69.

SkySports. *Sport England Slash Netball Funding.* 2014. http://www1.skysports.com/other-sports/news/12415/9235407/sport-england-slash-netball-funding (accessed December 10, 2014).

Slack, R., and P. Shrives. 'Beyond the Game. Perceptions and Practices of Corporate Social Responsibility in the Professional Sport Industry'. *Journal of Business Ethics* 91, no. 3 (2008): 433–50.

Smith, A., and H. Westerbeek. 'Sport as a Vehicle for Deploying Corporate Social Responsibility'. *Journal of Corporate Citizenship* 25 (2007): 43–54.

Weiss, C.H. 'Where Politics and Evaluation Research Meet'. *Evaluation Practice* 14, no. 1 (1993): 93–106.

Zwolinsky, S., J. McKenna, A. Pringle, and D. Parnell. 'Re: World Cup 2014: Festival of Football or Alcohol?' *BMJ: British Medical Journal* (2014): 348. doi:10.1136/bmj.g3772.

Index